# MAXIMISING ENERGY

Also by Suzannah Olivier

. . . . . . . . . . . . . . . . . . . . . . . . . . . . . . . . . . . . . . . . . .

Also in the *You Are What You Eat* series

. . . . . . . . . . . . . . . . . . . . . . . . . . . . . . . . . . . . . . . . . .

Suzannah Olivier

# MAXIMISING

# ENERGY

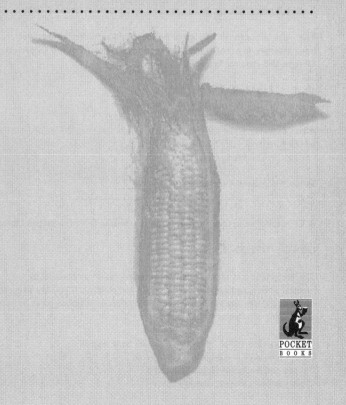

POCKET
BOOKS

First published in Great Britain by Pocket Books, 2000
An imprint of Simon & Schuster UK Ltd
A Viacom Company

10 9 8 7 6 5 4 3 2 1

Simon & Schuster UK Ltd
Africa House
64–78 Kingsway
London WC2B 6AH

Simon & Schuster Australia
Sydney

A CIP catalogue record for this book is available from the British Library

ISBN 0-671-02955-X

The information in this book is not intended as an alternative to
medical advice, and none of it is suitable for children. If you are pregnant, going
on an exclusion diet is not advised and professional advice must be sought
about using supplements and herbs.

Typeset in 12 on 14pt Perpetua with Gill Sans display
Design and page make-up by Peter Ward
Printed and bound in Great Britain by
Omnia Books Limited, Glasgow

Now I know how much energy is needed to raise kids,
I dedicate this book to my Mum.

# Contents

## TIRED ALL THE TIME

## APPENDICES

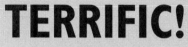

Part One

# ALL RIGHT ISN'T
# TERRIFIC!

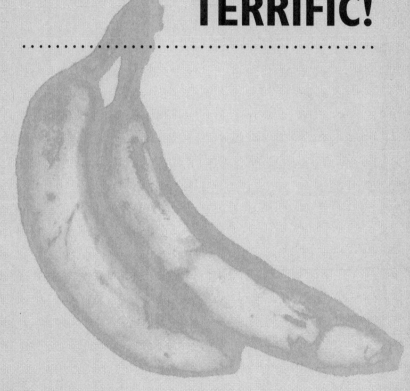

We all want more energy!

A lack of energy is one of the most common symptoms of impaired health and, although low energy is difficult to measure, you know when you are not reaching your full potential. And some people feel below par for months, or even years.

Most of us judge our level of energy by whether we feel awake when we get out of bed in the morning, and whether we have the stamina to carry us through our day. But there is a great deal more to energy than that. Not only does energy determine our ability to get up in the morning and get through the day, it also makes possible every process in our bodies – from the ability of our brains to think, to that of our guts to digest food, our hearts to beat and our lungs to breathe. In the course of a year over 90 per cent of your body will have renewed itself – the lining of the digestive tract in four days, your skin within six weeks, and even much of your bone tissue. While you are asleep your body isn't, and the stubble on a man's chin in the morning is evidence of this. Where is all this energy coming from, how do you create it, and is it possible to increase it?

Energy is not necessarily just the province of youth and aerobic fanatics, and those people who have boundless vitality are not merely lucky by chance. In reality there are quantifiable steps that can be taken to maximise the production of this seemingly elusive commodity. Energy doesn't just happen by some mysterious force. It is created in each and every cell day-in and day-out, as a result of 'fuel' being taken into our bodies, digested and metabolised.

Even if you are feeling OK, it is quite possible that you are not feeling as great as you might. We can't necessarily have it all, but we can all have some more. Quite a lot more, in fact.

## FALSE ENERGY

Many teenagers will be familiar with the scenario where they go clubbing all night, take assorted illicit substances to carry them through, and then roll into work the next day having had little or no sleep. So what has this got to do with you? The truth is that countless people live their lives in much the same way, but the difference is that the stimulants and drugs they use are totally legal, although still very addictive. Sugar and coffee, for example, fuel quick bursts of energy only to result in burn out later. Sugar and alcohol are sources of empty calories – calories which do not provide vitamins and minerals and, even worse, use up large amounts of these nutrients as the body attempts to deal with them. We are surrounded by these quick fixes, which give the illusion of energy, but in the long run deplete our resources and lead to flagging energy levels.

## BEING PUT ON NOTICE

When we experience an energy low, the temptation is often to just push through it and get on with whatever it is that needs doing. But early warning signs, such as extreme tiredness, are your body's way of telling you that you need to hold back for a while and regenerate. Ignore the warnings at your peril. Stressing your body leads to a number of common ailments – indigestion, headaches, migraines, thrush, eczema, arthritis, PMT, high blood pressure, eating disorders, depression, and so on.

When you are dealing with a crisis, say a viral infection, you have less net energy to, for example, wash the dishes, deal with the children, or file that report. Any stress on the body, whether it is physical, mental, emotional, or even nutritional, requires energy to deal with it – at the expense of energy being available for use elsewhere. In such circumstances, energy is diverted away from the ability to deal with daily tasks, and channelled into the tasks of healing, which is as it should be. But all too frequently we ignore this, pushing ourselves into an energy deficit, with the result that more and more people are visiting their GPs complaining that they feel constantly tired. This new syndrome has now been labelled TATT – tired all the time.

## GO FOR GOLD

No doubt some people do have the genetic predisposition to be more vital and energetic than the average person, and are able to do more before reaching the point at which they feel tired. We all know that some people thrive on four hours sleep a night, or are running marathons at the age of eighty, but what about mere mortals? Can you still maximise your potential energy levels? Undoubtedly you can. It is all a matter of achieving the right balance. By addressing your diet, and some lifestyle factors, you can improve your handling of stress, reduce your need to nap, become physically fitter and sharpen your mind. When you do feel tired it should be a 'healthy' tired, and not the type where you feel like a wrung-out dish-cloth.

### Tailoring your diet to suit your needs can

- increase energy levels
- improve mental clarity
- improve physical performance
- make your sleep more beneficial
- increase resistance to infections

# Part Two

# GENERATING

# ENERGY

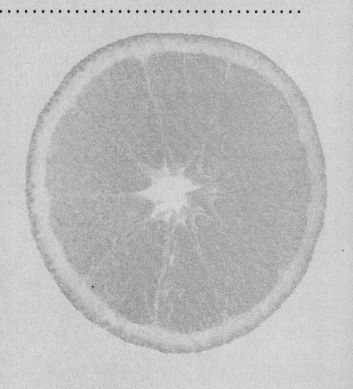

The way we generate energy is a fascinating process whereby the food we eat, and the air we breathe, is converted to power our body and mind.

Tiny 'organelles' (miniature organs called the mitochondria) in our cells act as energy factories. Inside these powerhouses, a carefully controlled sequence of reactions takes place, which manufactures energy. This sequence is called Kreb's cycle, after the man who first described it. During this process, our food is broken down and the carbohydrates end up as glucose. The glucose is then combusted with oxygen to produce units of energy in our cells called ATP. ATP is the currency of energy exchange within cells and is used to make muscles work, organs function and brain cells fire. The waste products of this amazing process are simply water and carbon dioxide.

How effective your body is at energy production largely depends on the quality of the raw materials used to stoke the fire. If you put logs on a fire it will burn steadily and give out a regular amount of heat. If you put newspaper on a fire it will burn furiously, and emit intense heat, but only for a short while before burning out. The quality of fuel you put into your body dictates how long-lasting your energy is.

We are capable of making energy from all three main components in our diet – proteins, fats and carbohydrates. But carbohydrates are the preferred source of fuel as they are the most clean burning. Carbohydrates are 'trapped energy', and they are made from the action of plants trapping energy from sunshine and storing it. When we eat plant foods we release that energy

for our own use. Proteins and fats are used, principally, for
building body tissues, and so are also important in determining
health. But if our bodies are forced to use proteins and fats, in
preference to carbohydrates, for energy production this results
in toxic by-products which need to be processed and eliminated. It is a little like adding rubber tyres to a fire – they will burn,
but give off toxic fumes at the same time.

## NUTRIENT-DENSE FOODS

In order for us to power the energy factories in each cell, we
need to provide them with the nutrients required for the whole
cycle to work. While carbohydrates, and sometimes fats and
proteins, provide the fuel, the 'fire-lighters', loosely-speaking,
are the vitamins and minerals (or micronutrients), as they
enable the whole process of metabolism to work. The most
important of these are the B-vitamins, vitamin C, magnesium,
zinc, iron, manganese and CoQ10.

The idea that a deficiency of some factor intrinsic to particular foods might be involved in fatigue was first suggested by Dr
James Lind, a ship's surgeon, in 1753. This was 150 years before
even the concept of vitamins was put forward! Dr Lind's *A
Treatise of Scurvy* reported the first ever controlled clinical trial
showing that citrus fruits were able to cure the disease. In it he
noted that the first symptom of scurvy was 'a listlessness to
action or an aversion to any sort of exercise . . . much fatigue
. . . breathlessness and panting'. He also noted that sailors who
were under stress developed scurvy faster than those who were
not, despite similar diets. We now know that the effects of stress
over a sustained period of time can cause us to use up to twice
the number of micronutrients we would use normally. Modern
studies have since shown that there is a significant relationship
between vitamin C intake – the substance in the citrus fruit that

reversed the scurvy Dr Lind was commenting on – and general fatigue. We also now know that this relationship also holds true for a number of other nutrients.

It is absolutely essential for the whole process of energy creation that we eat energy- and nutrient-dense foods. Nature is ingenious and has given us foods which are rich in the nutrients needed to process and metabolise them. The food processing industry, on the other hand, has managed to create a massive supply of convenience foods, and stimulants, which have few intrinsic nutrients. These foods are the 'poor relations' of more natural foods, since although they are sources of calories, or energy, they are not nutrient-dense and lack vitamins, minerals and fibre. The nutrients have been stripped out of them during processing and, with few exceptions, have not been added back in again. Even when they have, as in the case of bread and cereals, it is usually only a selection of nutrients that has been added back in, and not all of them. As a result, our diets are sadly deficient in many of the essential nutrients.

According to the latest available UK Government figures average diets fail to meet the RNIs (Recommended Nutrient Intakes) as follows:

| | Men | Women |
| --- | --- | --- |
| vitamin A | 27% | 31% |
| vitamin B2 | 12% | 21% |
| vitamin B6 | 6% | 22% |
| vitamin B12* | 1% | 4% |
| folic acid | 12% | 47% |
| vitamin C | 26% | 34% |
| calcium | 25% | 48% |
| copper** | 24% | 59% |
| iodine | 9% | 32% |

| | Men | Women |
|---|---|---|
| iron | 12% | 89% |
| magnesium | 42% | 72% |
| potassium | 65% | 94% |
| zinc | 31% | 31% |

*While dietary intake seems more or less acceptable for a majority of people, problems with absorption suggest that a significant number of people may be deficient, see Anaemia page 108.

**While dietary intake of copper may be low, it is likely that a significant number of people have excessively high blood levels due to contamination of water supplies and use of the Pill and HRT (hormone replacement therapy). High copper levels interfere with the uptake of zinc and iron.

Some of the figures on this chart become even more shocking when you begin to look at them in more detail. For example, the RNI for vitamin C is a paltry 40 mg, the amount you would get in two thirds of an orange. This means that a quarter to one third of the population are not getting even this! I began this section by talking about vitamin C and scurvy, a disease one would have thought was consigned to the history books, and of passing interest only. Indeed this is the way it is taught in medical schools. And yet in the last ten years doctors have seen a recurrence of scurvy because of the lamentable quality of the foods which make up our diets.

Some foods are so over-processed that they provide 'empty calories', notably sugar and alcohol, which have been totally stripped of all the vitamins and nutrients that are needed to metabolise them. For instance, molasses, which is the residue left behind when sugar is made, is higher in calcium, and other minerals, weight for weight, than milk. And yet sugar has none of the co-factors left in it to enable us to process it. The stress caused by this on the body is considerable, and a great drain on stored nutrient reserves. A good example of this is the mineral chromium. Sugar causes a net loss of this mineral as it is excreted in the urine after eating sugar. This can lead to sugar-handling problems because chromium is vital for processing sugar.

In order to ensure a diet which is nutrient-dense, it is necessary to eat foods that are as unadulterated as possible. A banana-flavoured instant pudding, for example, contains virtually no nutrients apart from the milk used to make it up. A banana mashed with plain yoghurt, on the other hand, with some added chopped nuts, will be nutrient-dense. A coffee and doughnut provides virtually no nutrients (and causes a net loss of them), but an oat flapjack eaten with a glass of fresh juice will be nutrient-packed. A jam sandwich made with white bread has a much reduced nutritive value compared to a peanut butter or avocado sandwich on wholemeal bread, which will give a nutrient boost. It is all about making educated choices. A diet which is rich in wholegrains, pulses, vegetables, fruits, fresh nuts and seeds, contains moderate amounts of dairy products and meat, and which avoids refined foods, is a nutrient-rich diet.

## THE ENERGY SPIRAL

From the moment we put food into our mouths our system works hard to break it down into its smallest and simplest components in order that it can be used for building blocks or for energy production. As already mentioned, carbohydrates are the primary source of fuel for the thousands of body processes, and all the carbohydrates we eat, refined or complex, are turned into glucose in our blood. No matter what foods they come from, this is the fate of carbohydrates. The glucose in the blood triggers the hormone insulin to be secreted by the pancreas, and it is insulin which is needed to get carbohydrates, as well as fats and proteins, into the cells to be used for energy. Surplus glucose which is not used immediately for energy is stored as short-term energy reserves – as glycogen – in the muscles or in the liver. If the glycogen is not used within a short time, because we are insufficiently active, or we have too much glycogen being built up, it is stored as long-term 'potential' energy, as fat.

Despite all carbohydrates being made from glucose units, and having the potential to break down into glucose in the blood, they are not all created equal. What is relevant to the energy equation is how fast – or more to the point how slowly – they break down into glucose. For the most part sugar, foods high in sugars and refined carbohydrates – as listed in the chart below – break down quickly into glucose. If this surprises you, there is a simple test you can do to get an idea of just how quickly the process takes effect. Take a small piece of white bread and keep it in your mouth for a minute or so. (We have carbohydrate splitting enzymes in the saliva in our mouth.) You will find that quite quickly the bread begins to break down into sugars, and that it becomes sweet tasting.

Humans are carbohydrate eaters and this is why we have a naturally sweet tooth. When we are babies our first encounter with sweet carbohydrates comes from breast milk and the milk sugars in mothers' milk is extremely sweet! However, most carbohydrate foods found in nature are slow-releasing. The exception to this is honey, a delight to which our ancestors did not have easy access – it did not come out of a jar! The most abundant sugar, and a direct source of fuel, was fructose, the slow-releasing sugar found in fruit. Since we are not designed to deal with large amounts of fast-releasing carbohydrates, our blood sugar levels, if we do succumb to them, go haywire in an attempt to regulate the situation.

Carbohydrates come in several shapes and sizes. Examples of the simplest sugars are the single molecules of glucose or fructose. Next in complexity are the sugars which link two molecules together, the disaccharides, such as sucrose (table sugar), lactose (milk sugar) and maltose. The next most complex carbohydrates are the starches, which link many molecules together in pearl necklace-like strands, or in a branched arrangement like a tree.

Previous dietary advice to diabetics who needed to control their blood sugar levels was to avoid sugar and eat everything else. And yet sugar releases energy at about the same rate as bread. And while it is generally true to say that sugars can be considered fast-releasing, fructose, which is fruit sugar, is particularly slow-releasing, despite being one of the simplest sugars. It is now obvious that the effect of different foods on blood sugar balance is more complex than was once thought, and we are only now just beginning to understand what these effects are.

## Sources of fast-releasing carbohydrates

sugar

honey

some dried fruit (dates, raisins, figs)

some vegetables (cooked root vegetables: potato, beets, parsnips, carrots, swede)

milk (lactose milk sugar)

many processed grains (bread, rice, some pasta, corn)

## Sources of slow-releasing carbohydrates

most whole grains

beans, peas, lentils

most fruits and fructose (fruit sugar)

most vegetables

If your diet consists predominantly of foods from the first list, then you are getting a lot of quick-releasing sugars into your system. These sugars give a quick 'hit' of energy, but they are stressful for the body's regulatory systems to deal with. Boosts of sugars and other fast-releasing carbohydrates over-stimulate the pancreas to produce insulin, with the result that blood sugar levels can then come crashing down as the insulin overcompensates for the excess sugar. This causes a blood sugar low, as there is now insufficient glucose in the blood to carry out normal functions efficiently.

## SYMPTOMS OF BLOOD SUGAR IMBALANCE

Glucose is used for all body functions, including brain function. The brain, which accounts for only around 5 per cent of body weight, is so energy hungry that, even when at rest, it uses up at least 30 per cent of available glucose, and the brain and nervous system are acutely sensitive to fluctuations in blood sugar levels. The result is that when you experience a blood sugar low you may experience 'brain fag' as well as low physical reserves. The message your body usually sends you, loud and clear, is 'I want you to lie down – now'. To overcome this, what do most people do? They override the message by having another quick hit of a sugary food, or other stimulant. This creates spirals of energy highs and lows. The momentum becomes increasingly difficult to maintain and eventually, when an individual's physical reserves are too depleted, can lead to more serious exhaustion.

If this occurs, and blood sugar levels fall too far and too rapidly, the symptoms, which are the result of adrenaline emergency hormone output, can include sweating, weakness, hunger, rapid heart beat and feelings of anxiety. If blood sugar levels drop more slowly, but still too far, the symptoms, over a period of time, could include headaches, blurred vision, double vision, mental confusion and incoherent speech. If low blood sugar levels then persist over a period of hours possible symptoms can include outbursts of temper, depression, prolonged sleepiness and restlessness. Added to these classical symptoms of low blood sugar are many other symptoms of conditions that are linked to the problem, including light-headedness, addictions, alcoholism, arthritis, food allergies, insomnia, frequent nightmares, migraine headaches and high IQ children labelled as under-achievers or hyperactive.

## Are You Affected by Blood Sugar Lows?

1 Do you have less energy than you used to?
2 Are you slow to get going in the morning?
3 Do you often feel drowsy during the day time?
4 Do you avoid exercise due to lack of energy?
5 Are you affected by mood swings?
6 Do you feel as if you are under constant stress?
7 Are you affected by poor concentration?
8 Do you need something to get you going in the morning (tea, coffee, sugar, cigarette)?
9 Do you need energy 'props' throughout the day (tea, coffee, sugar, cigarettes, alcohol)?
10 Do you get dizzy or irritable if you don't eat for six hours?

### Scoring:

**0–2** Your blood sugar levels are probably reasonably balanced. If you are lacking in energy it may be due to other factors such as overwork, sleeping patterns or stress.

**3–4** You are showing signs of blood sugar imbalance and addressing this is likely to lead to significant improvements. You may find that this is the only issue you need to address to improve your energy levels.

**5–7** Your score is getting quite high and you need to address blood sugar as a matter of priority. It is likely that you will find that other hormonal imbalances are contributing to your problems and you may need to address other issues, such as stress (adrenal function), thyroid function or food addictions.

**8–10** Your score indicates blood sugar imbalance that may be quite debilitating. Addressing blood sugar problems is a necessity in your case. If your symptoms are accompanied by excessive thirst, frequent urination and 'sweet' breath you are best advised to have a urine test at your doctor's surgery to ensure that you are not edging towards diabetes.

It is not just one sugary meal or snack that has a detrimental effect, but the cumulative effect of eating this way day-in, day-out, often since childhood, that leads to problems with the ability to regulate blood sugar levels. By changing your diet, you can feel the benefits of balanced blood sugar in a fairly short period of time. Within a couple of weeks you can benefit from more energy, less drowsiness and more balanced moods. This is because your blood sugar graph looks like this:

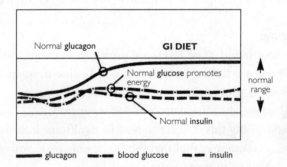

Instead
of this:

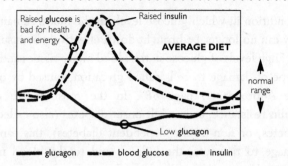

Raised **glucose** is
bad for health
and energy

Raised **insulin**

**AVERAGE DIET**

normal
range

Low **glucagon**

━━━ glucagon   ━━▪━━ blood glucose   ━━ ━━ insulin

Spot the difference? What is happening in the second illustration is that insulin is overcorrecting, and removing glucose too rapidly from the bloodstream, causing blood sugar to crash to a level well below what it was at prior to eating.

If you alter the type of carbohydrates you eat you will notice significant benefits in your energy levels within a few weeks. Hopefully, this improvement will then motivate you to continue in this way for life.

## SYNDROME X

Some people, who may be genetically susceptible, progress a stage further with their blood sugar problems, and the scales tip over into a condition known as insulin resistance. In such people, insulin is produced as normal, but the body's cells are resistant to its effects. This means that the level of glucose in their blood remains high as it has nowhere to go.

The phenomenon of high insulin levels has been termed syndrome X, and it is implicated in raised blood pressure (50 per cent of patients with high blood pressure have insulin resistance), poor cholesterol levels and raised blood fats (triglycerides), and inflammatory diseases. The effort of maintaining insulin levels probably leads to 'burn out' of the insulin producing cells in the pancreas, and can result in adult-onset diabetes, a condition in which glucose levels in the blood remain high as they can no longer be brought down effectively by insulin.

High levels of glucose in the blood injure tissues and leads to a type of damage to cells called glycation, caused by oxidation (see **Antioxidants**, page 58). In the most severe cases of insulin resistance, as in adult onset diabetes (also called Type II diabetes, or non-insulin dependent diabetes), this can lead to damage to the eyes, the kidneys and to the blood network. Recent, large-scale, studies have shown that diabetics who keep their blood sugar under tight control can largely avoid the complications of this disease. The incidence of diabetes has risen sharply in the last fifteen years. Two per cent of the population are now affected, and 10 per cent of the NHS budget is currently devoted to its management.

The absence of diabetes in populations where no refined foods are eaten confirm that diet is the main factor involved. While some people may be genetically more susceptible to the problem, this is not the whole answer, and diet is the most powerful way of avoiding it. This is best illustrated when you look at how diabetic strains of rats are bred for laboratories. Rats are fed sugar to make them diabetic, and are then mated with other sugar-induced diabetic rats. The result is a diabetic strain. Unwittingly, humans following the typical diet found in the UK and USA have been subject to exactly the same experiment on a massive scale. Until very recently we did not eat sugar or refined foods, and yet today 20 to 25 per cent of our diet is derived from sugars, which have displaced other foods, such as fruits, vegetables and whole grains. We now eat between 45–65 kg of sugar annually per person, and 80 per cent of that sugar comes from processed and packaged foods.

Insulin resistance may well be a significant factor in those who complain of TATT (tired all the time), as according to Dr Reaven, a leading US authority in the field, it is seen in around

25 per cent of the population. He found that 'Insulin resistance is present in a majority of patients with impaired glucose tolerance (blood sugar balance) or non-insulin dependent diabetes, and in approximately 25 per cent of non-obese individuals with normal glucose tolerance'. Other researchers have backed up his findings. They also suggest that being obese significantly increases the risk of having problems with insulin resistance, although as many as one in four normal weight people are also insulin resistant.

## STRESS AND BLOOD SUGAR

Stress is a major player in the blood sugar picture. The tiny glands which govern our response to stress are the adrenal glands, which sit like hats on top of our kidneys. They produce a number of hormones, including the stress hormones adrenaline, noradrenaline and cortisol. Between them these hormones are responsible for coping with short-term acute stress and longer-term chronic stress.

Humans, along with all mammals, produce a quick shot of adrenaline if we are put under stress, a phenomenon named as the 'fight or flight syndrome' by Hans Selyé in the 1930s. What he meant by this was that, when faced with an emergency – which in evolutionary terms is usually thought of as being attacked by a predator – we would summon up the reserves to 'fight' or 'flee'. Within seconds of being faced with a threat – which in today's terms might be stopping a child running out into the road – our heart is pounding, muscles tense, eyes dilate, breathing changes, the hairs on our body stand on end and our blood thickens. This response is dependent on access to an instant reserve of energy, in the form of glucose, and we conjure this up from our stores of readily available energy, glycogen, which is stored in readiness in muscles and in the liver.

Adrenaline is the means by which we access this, as one of its chief effects is to liberate, in an instant, glucose from glycogen stores to raise blood sugar levels. Apart from food intake, adrenaline is therefore the most important means by which blood sugar levels are raised. This is fine, and indeed necessary, if we are in an emergency, but thankfully most of us do not live on the edge of crisis all the time.

What is more common, is a low-level of constant stress, which keeps our stress hormone levels inappropriately high over long periods. Astoundingly, the adrenaline rush of the average commuter stuck in a traffic jam is enough to keep them running for a mile. This can be extremely disruptive to blood sugar levels.

## ADDICTIVE STIMULANTS

Adding to this effect are the many stimulants to which we seem, as a society, to be addicted. A shot of coffee, or a single cigarette will not, in themselves, cause a crisis, although they will trigger adrenaline at the time. What is a problem, however, is perpetual exposure to a number of stimulants and relaxants. You may think that you are quite moderate but the following is a typical, and moderate, day for many people. The cumulative effect is that blood sugar levels are being kept abnormally high.

> 2 cups of coffee in the morning
> 4 cups of tea during the day
> biscuits or a bag of crisps mid-morning
> a chocolate bar mid-afternoon
> 2 alcoholic drinks during the evening

This adds up to ten occasions during the day that blood sugar is being triggered. Ten times a day, means seventy times a week, equals 3,650 times a year. Put in such a way, you can see why the real problem is the cumulative effect. And, to reiterate, most people would think this was quite moderate. It does not, for example, take into account any cigarettes smoked or the effects on adrenaline that food sensitivities (or more accurately addictions) will have, as they also throw the body into crisis. You will know if this applies to you if, for instance, you can't get through the day without bread (this is discussed in more detail in **Throw Away The Crutches**, page 38).

At this stage you could start making a daily note, for a week, of all the times you consume foods or drinks, or do anything else, which might cause your blood sugar to rise. At the end of the week you will be able to see if any pattern has emerged. You should note intake of any of the following:

- coffee
- cigarettes
- strong tea
- sugar or sugary food
- chocolate
- alcohol
- any food you are eating because of comfort/addiction (usually carbohydrates such as potatoes, bread, rice, pasta, biscuits, potato crisps or cheese)
- intense exercise which gives you a 'high'
- stressful situations (either 'positive' stress or 'negative' stress)
- any other stimulants, including 'psychological stimulants' such as a dangerous sport
- recreational drugs

## OUR ABILITY TO ADAPT

Hans Selyé also coined the term 'general adaptive syndrome' (GAS). What he meant by this is that we have the most tremen-

dous ability to adapt to our surroundings and circumstances in
the short term. This is one of the factors that has made us so successful as a species. Selyé suggested that, when we are faced with
a new stressor, we go through three stages: the alarm phase, the
adaptive phase and the exhaustion stage. There also seems to be
a fourth stage – the hypersensitivity stage.

For instance, if you take the case of coffee, cast your mind
back to the first time you tasted it. It is largely an acquired taste
and most children will shy away from it. The first cup you had
probably gave you quite a buzz. This buzz was the alarm phase,
when the substance, coffee in this case, had a strong effect. The
same would be true of the first cigarette (coughing and a sore
throat), alcohol (light-headedness). The next stage is the
adaptation stage, when you acclimatise to the substance, and
eventually find that you need more of it to get the same effect.
So your occasional coffee goes up to several cups a day. During
this phase there is a price to pay. For example, coffee, if drunk
to calm nerves at a stressful moment, will trigger stress
hormones to a greater degree than the stress alone would do.
High levels of coffee intake will, along with other stressors, have
a significant effect on the adrenal glands, and can help to push
you over the edge into exhaustion. This is the exhaustion stage.
So you give up coffee, and address stress and dietary issues and
return to even health. This is where the fourth possible stage
comes in. Many people will then become hypersensitive to
whatever it is that was involved in the stress reaction. One cup
of coffee now may be enough to give you the shakes or keep you
awake all night. What you are experiencing is the initial response
again. The effect can be quite pronounced, with a pounding
head, a racing mind, a speeded up heart beat and, possibly,
drowsiness, as your blood sugar levels plummet again. You may
also have experienced withdrawal headaches at the point when

you gave up the coffee, giving you an idea of just how much of a drug it is.

You can follow this scenario through with most stressors, and it can be quite illuminating to think about events in your life that have mirrored this pattern. For instance, the person who overworks and then becomes workshy, the smoker who won't go into a room where people are smoking, and so on. I'm sure you can think of examples that relate to you.

# Part Three

# EATING FOR

# ENERGY

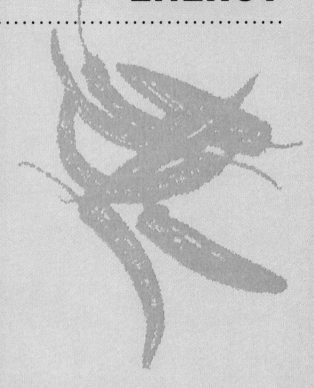

## THE GI DIET

The glycaemic index (GI) measures the speed with which carbohydrate foods affect blood sugar levels. The most important principle to adhere to when trying to maximise energy levels is to choose foods which appear low down on the GI chart, and to restrict or avoid foods which score highly.

By following this advice, you can also reduce cravings for particular foods, and the need to overeat, since high GI foods have been shown to increase appetite, which, in turn, leads to the craving to eat more of these carbohydrate foods, perpetuating the downward spiral. One interesting study gave two groups of people 200 calories of sugar to eat before letting them loose, two hours later, on a banquet at which they could eat as much as they wanted. One of the groups ate an average of 476 calories less than the other. What was the difference? The sugar that was given to the group who ate less calories was fructose (fruit sugar), which has a very low GI of 22, while the other group were given glucose, which has a GI of 100. This probably accounts for why, a couple of hours after eating a filling Chinese meal, people often complain that they are hungry – rice and noodles have relatively high GI. Other studies have backed this up. In one, obese teenage boys were given one of three breakfasts – a high GI meal of instant oatmeal, a medium GI meal of whole oats, or a low GI meal of a vegetable omelette and fruit. Later in the day the voluntary calorie intake after the high GI meal was 53 per cent greater than it was for the medium GI meal, and 81 per cent more than after the low GI meal.

This is an abbreviated GI chart for quick reference, but for a full chart see **Appendix II**, page 142.

| High GI 71–100 Restrict | | Medium GI 51–70 Moderate | | Low GI 15–50 Enjoy | |
|---|---|---|---|---|---|
| sultana bran | 71 | orange juice | 52 | yoghurt, low fat | 14 |
| puffed wheat | 74 | kiwi fruit | 53 | fructose | 22 |
| pumpkin | 75 | sweet potato | 54 | 70% cocoa solids | |
| chips | 75 | banana | 54 | chocolate | 22 |
| doughnut | 76 | sweetcorn | 55 | full fat milk | 27 |
| rice cakes | 77 | oatmeal biscuits | 55 | lentils | 29 |
| vanilla wafers | 77 | buckwheat | 55 | butter beans | 31 |
| plain biscuits | 77 | durum wheat | | dried apricots | 31 |
| white bread | 78 | spaghetti | 55 | skimmed milk | 32 |
| broad beans | 79 | muesli | 56 | pear | 37 |
| jelly beans | 80 | mango | 56 | whole-wheat | |
| rice crispies/corn- | | Kelloggs Mini- | | spaghetti | 37 |
| flakes | 82 | wheats | 57 | apple | 38 |
| baked potato | | honey | 58 | plum | 39 |
| (old potato) | 85 | porridge (oatmeal) | 61 | All-bran | 42 |
| cooked carrots | 85 | beetroot | 64 | orange | 44 |
| Lucozade | 95 | sucrose | 64 | chickpeas | 45 |
| French baguette | 95 | raisins | 64 | Yakult | 45 |
| parsnips | 97 | high fibre rye | | grapefruit juice | 48 |
| dates | 99 | crispbreads | 65 | baked beans | 48 |
| glucose | 100 | Grapenuts | 66 | peas, green | 48 |
| maltodextrin | 105 | Nutri-grain | 66 | raw carrots | 49 |
| maltose | 105 | pineapple | 66 | pumpernickel bread | 50 |
| | | mashed potato | 70 | | |

What influences the effect that foods have in GI terms is quite complex, being a sum of the types of carbohydrates, combined with the fibre content, the protein content and the fat content. The GI was developed in 1981, but it is only in very recent years that we have come to fully understand the effects that individual foods have within the context of the whole diet. For the most part, the foods which have a swift impact on blood sugar levels and score highest are fairly obvious, such as most sugars. But there are some surprises, such as potatoes, carrots, pizza and maltodextrine (a processed starch used in vast quantities by the food industry which appears in many packaged foods). Potatoes have a GI similar to that of sugar. Does that make them a bad food? If you are prone to energy and blood sugar problems then they are best moderated, for others, however, they are a valuable source of nutrients, while sugar is simply a source of empty calories, with no nutrients, and is best limited by everyone.

There are also differences in grains. Those high in a starch called amylopectin, such as wheat, corn and most types of rice, are faster-releasing than those high in the starch amylose, such as barley, rye, quinoa and brown basmati rice. A pleasant surprise is barley, which is one of the lowest-scoring GI grains. It cooks like rice, making it an easy, and delicious, substitute. One reason why legume foods, such as lentils and soya, are so low down on the scale is that they contain a substance which slows the digestion of amylose and so reduces further its impact on insulin.

The processing of foods makes a difference, too. If you take a bag of wheat and turn it into pasta, it will have a lower GI than if you turn it into bread. Studies have shown that the scores for wheat, corn and oats increase when they go from the whole grain, to cracked grains, to coarse flour to finely ground flour – and the grains used were not refined ones, stripped of fibre and nutrients, but simply increasingly ground grains. The GI concerns itself with averages because an under-ripe banana, for example, scores 30, making it a low-GI food, whereas a ripe banana scores 54, making it a medium-GI food. The reason for this is that, when under-ripe, 80–90 per cent of a banana's carbohydrate content is starch, but as it ripens this changes to free sugars. Depending on the type, the starch content of rice ranges from 38–93 per cent, and that of potatoes from 47–95 per cent.

Fruits and vegetables have different effects depending on their sugar make up. Fruits which contain higher amounts of fructose (fruit sugar) have a slowish effect on blood sugar, as it needs to be converted into glucose. However, some fruits contain significant amounts of glucose along with the fructose. These include grapes, pineapples, watermelon and very ripe bananas. This means that a banana might be a good option if you have just been jogging and need a glucose top-up, but if you have blood sugar problems it may give you too quick a 'hit'. This does not make bananas a bad food, but you would be best combining them with, for instance, porridge oats to slow down their impact. An even better option would be to have grated apple with the porridge. You may find that so called 'sugar-free' foods are sweetened with grape juice, which is tantamount to adding glucose, while others use apple juice, which does not have such a direct effect on blood sugar.

There are also differences in different brands of certain foods. The manufacturing process can cause significant differences in the carbohydrate content of different soya milks. Depending on whether they are unsweetened or sweetened they can range from 4–36 grams of carbohydrates per 225 ml/8 fl oz of product. This will affect the GI score. Dairy milk ranges between 11–13 grams of carbohydrates per 225 ml/8 fl oz, however the lactose found in it has a higher GI than the carbohydrates found in soya milk.

Vegetables can also spring a surprise in the blood sugar control stakes. Most are very low on the glycaemic index, and as a result are to be encouraged as the mainstay of most meals (I know, you are saying, 'Yummy, spinach for breakfast!'). However, most root vegetables quickly turn into sugars when they are cooked. The best illustration of this is the fact that much of the world's supply of sugar comes from sugar beet, which is a type of beetroot. When you bake carrots or parsnips they caramelise easily, making you realise just how sweet they are.

Once you understand the basics of the way in which the GI diet works you can make some easy choices to balance your blood sugar levels. Here are some of them:

| Instead of Fast-releasing GI Foods | Choose Slow-releasing GI Foods |
| --- | --- |
| white bread, 'brown' bread* | wholegrain rye bread |
| white rice | brown basmati rice, barley, Quinoa |
| rice cakes | rye crackers, oat cakes |
| cornflakes, rice puffs | porridge, muesli, All-bran |
| jam | 100% fruit jam, nut butters |
| cooked parsnips, carrots, beets, potatoes or swede | cooked yams, sweet potatoes, or corn (mid GI) raw root vegetables, butter beans, flageolet beans, peas |
| dates | dried apricots, dried apple rings, fresh fruit |
| milk chocolate | 70% cocoa solids chocolate |

* 'Brown' bread is very often the equivalent of white bread 'coloured' brown, unless it is labelled wholemeal, wholegrain or wholewheat.

## TOTAL MEAL EFFECT

Choosing foods which appear low down on the GI is the first place to start if you want sustained energy. However, it is also necessary to remember that the total meal combination – in other words the balance of proteins and fats to carbohydrates on your plate – affects blood sugar balance.

To refresh your memory, insulin is the hormone that lowers blood sugar, while glucagon is the one that raises it, and it is a balance between these two that is sought. Carbohydrate foods eaten on their own, especially fast-releasing ones, result in a large insulin response and a small glucagon release.

When eaten on their own, protein foods tend to result in a small and equal release of insulin and glucagon. This means that they have little direct impact on blood sugar levels. However, if they are eaten alongside carbohydrates, they slightly temper the effect that carbohydrates have on insulin.

Eating fats on their own has no direct impact on either hormone, but they do slow down the effect that carbohydrates have on insulin. Some 'sinful' foods seem tantalisingly acceptable on the GI, but this is due to their fat content. For instance, Mars Bars, which contain an average nine teaspoons of sugar, are tempered in their effect by their high fat content. Crisps, which are made from potato flour, would normally be around 95 on the GI, but are lower because they are so high in fat. This does not make them 'good' foods. Pizzas remain an anomaly, and have been shown in research to have a more dramatic impact on blood sugar than would be expected. Like other high scoring GI foods, pizzas trigger a high initial response, but, unlike other foods, they continue to create this response after the blood levels caused by eating comparable foods begin to decline. Pity the poor pizza eaters!

The effects of the various elements of our diet on insulin and glucose are as follows:

| | Insulin | Glucagon |
|---|---|---|
| carbohydrate | ***** | no change |
| protein | ** | ** |
| fat | no change | no change |
| carbohydrate and fat | **** | no change |
| protein and fat | ** | * |
| high protein and low carbohydrate | ** | * |
| high carbohydrate and low protein | ***** | * |

* = small effect  ***** = strong effect (with sliding scale in between)

Quite a number of people follow the principles of 'food combining', otherwise known as the Hay diet, where they do not mix 'dense' proteins and 'dense' carbohydrates at the same meal ('dense' meaning that the food consists of more than 80 per cent protein or carbohydrate). While this way of eating is highly beneficial for people with digestive problems, it is not the way to balance blood sugar levels. You can see from the above chart that eating carbohydrates on their own, or carbohydrates with a minimal amount of protein, would release a large amount of insulin with little opposing glucagon. Following the Hay diet, and eating such meals twice a day, would undoubtedly exacerbate insulin resistance in susceptible people. For this reason, it is best to eat some protein alongside carbohydrates at each meal to stabilise blood sugar levels. The food combining principle can achieve this if adherents eat meals consisting of a little protein, such as fish, chicken, eggs, meat or soya foods, alongside a lot of vegetables. However, if the food combining follower ends up eating meals that are heavily biased towards 'dense' carbohydrates, such as rice, pasta or bread, with no protein to balance them, then this can play havoc with blood sugar levels, and therefore energy levels.

Eating meals which combine carbohydrates and proteins has also been shown to be the best support for the stress/adrenal system. Because of the critical part that the adrenal hormone system plays in maintaining energy levels this is another reason to favour this way of eating if your energy levels are flagging. For the best effect, the important thing is to eat low GI foods – vegetables, fruits, pulses, beans, soya, and some grains, such as rye and barley – alongside proteins.

## FREQUENCY OF EATING

While aiming to stabilise blood sugar levels it is important to pre-empt the possibility of blood sugar lows. The way to do this is to eat small, frequent meals. This does not necessarily mean eating more, but it does help if you can spread out your food intake over five or six small meals instead of eating two or three large ones. By doing this, and by making sure that the snacks are those which do not have a negative effect on blood sugar balance, you can significantly increase your energy levels. It is common for busy people to skip breakfast, or even for people to believe that they are not hungry at this time, and this is the first major mistake that is made. It is also often the case that morning hunger signals are over-ridden by a cup of strong coffee. After ten to twelve hours without food your body needs fuel and it is no wonder that skipping breakfast is the first step in ensuring that blood sugar levels swing up and down wildly all day. Even if you are in a rush, you have time to grab a couple of pieces of fruit, a small yoghurt and some oatcakes, and if necessary take them with you.

## MORE THAN JUST BLOOD SUGAR LEVELS

High GI foods do not just dent your energy levels. They also activate more insulin, which activates a substance called HMACoA reductase, which causes the liver to make more cholesterol. In this way high GI foods, and other blood sugar triggering substances such as alcohol, indirectly influence cholesterol levels. Low GI foods have been shown to promote 'healthy' HDL cholesterol over 'unhealthy' LDL cholesterol. Because high GI foods play havoc with blood sugar control, this leads to increased oxidation damage to tissues, including those in the arteries. This helps explain the relationship between syndrome X and the risk of heart disease.

And believe it or not, if you eat non-refined foods, you will also be contributing to the health of the planet, as well as your own, by maximising energy resources. Processing a golden field of wheat into a sugary breakfast cereal takes considerably more energy than turning it into wholewheat bread. If everyone switched their diets towards unrefined foods the energy savings would be huge.

## A SUMMARY OF HOW TO ADDRESS BLOOD SUGAR PROBLEMS WITH DIET

The way to regulate blood sugar levels is to eat little and often in order to pre-empt a blood sugar low. It is also necessary to avoid foods that are converted too quickly into glucose, and to concentrate on eating those that are rich in starches, or complex carbohydrates. It also helps to have some proteins alongside the carbohydrates.

The ideal is to eat three moderate meals, plus two between-meal snacks, and another before bedtime. The main points are:

I    Meals need to be eaten on time to avoid blood sugar lows and to maintain energy levels. Do not skip breakfast.

**2**    Snacks are essential to keep sugar levels constant as they maintain the necessary level of fuel and nutrients.

**3**    Eat foods that release their fuel slowly – these are principally fibre-rich carbohydrates, such as fruit, vegetables, pulses, legumes and some grains, such as rye and barley – along with proteins.

**5**    Avoid eating energy consumers. These are refined carbohydrates, processed foods, caffeine and other stimulants.

For serving suggestions see **Menu Plans**, page 69.

## THROW AWAY THE CRUTCHES

Energy props can be likened to filling a petrol tank with rocket fuel. All they do is provide a short burst of energy, which burns out just as fast. Stimulants may seem to give you a terrific boost, but they are the easiest way of draining your body of energy in the long run. Not only do they not provide consistent fuel, they also use up nutrients by the bucketful. By surviving on foods that are depleted of nutrients, and the source of 'empty calories', we miss out on the opportunity to nourish ourselves and to provide our energy manufacturing system with the basic tools it needs to do its job.

Legal stimulants include coffee, which contains a cocktail of chemicals called the methylxanthines (caffeine, theobromine and theophylline), strong tea, which contains caffeine, cola drinks (including some energy and sports drinks), which contain caffeine, cigarettes, which contains nicotine, and chocolate, which contains caffeine and theophylline. Add to this demanding jobs, horror movies, thrillers, emotional traumas and stressful news in the papers and on television, and you can see why it becomes increasingly difficult to relax while living on stimulants. We need more and more of them to get through the day, and because relaxing eventually becomes so difficult, we then learn to use other crutches – alcohol, sleeping pills, antidepressants, cannabis and the like.

Convincing yourself that you don't need the crutches is often more difficult than getting by without them. The leap of faith required may seem too great, but the truth is that you do not need stimulants, or relaxants. Most animals do not need a cup of coffee to get them through the day. I say most, because if they are introduced to stimulants in controlled laboratory experiments, they too become dependent on them. There is also evidence of some animals nibbling on leaves that have pharmacological properties – in other words they get high! We have learned from all these animals that it is easy to get addicted to various substances, and we know from our own experiences that this is true.

## STIMULANTS AFFECT BRAIN CHEMICALS

There are a number of brain chemicals that affect how we feel, and it is the reactions of these brain chemicals to certain foods and stimulants that makes them so addictive. The main ones to consider are serotonin, beta-endorphins and dopamine.

Serotonin levels are important in determining our moods and whether we feel satisfied when we eat. A correct level of this vital brain chemical is mood-stabilising. We make serotonin, our 'satisfaction' brain chemical, from an amino acid (protein link) called L-tryptophan, which is found in foods such as fish, turkey, chicken, pheasant, partridge, cottage cheese, beef, eggs, bananas, wheat germ, oats, avocados, milk, cheese, nuts, peanuts, soya beans, baked beans, sweet potato, alfalfa, beetroot, Brussels sprouts, carrots, cauliflower, celery, chives, fennel, spinach and watercress. In order to encourage the L-tryptophan to convert into serotonin it is important to eat carbohydrates alongside these proteins. We have already discussed the benefits of combining protein with slow-releasing carbohydrates to obtain steady energy levels, so this is another reason why eating these foods together can benefit health.

If levels of serotonin are low, we can be tempted to reach for foods that lift our spirits and give us a serotonin boost, and sugary and refined carbohydrate foods, as well as alcohol, will do just that. True to anything with addictive qualities, however, these foods only make us feel good in the short term. This, of course, leads to a vicious cycle of sugar and refined carbohydrate cravings which perpetuates the problem of serotonin imbalance.

The same thing occurs, more or less, with beta-endorphins, where sugar and alcohol act to increase the levels. Beta-endorphins are 'pleasure' brain chemicals, which have a similar action to the opiate drugs morphine and heroin. Interestingly, wheat and dairy products, the foods that are most commonly addictive, and which cause the most sensitivity problems, also appear to have an opiate effect. Beta-endorphin levels are lower premenstrually, which may explain why cravings for sugary foods tends to increase at this time (blood sugar levels are also more temperamental at this time).

Dopamine is another brain chemical, made from the amino acid L-tyrosine. Sugar, alcohol and coffee stimulate the production of dopamine, but, once again, they provide only a short term mood boost, the penalty being that you soon feel the effect of low dopamine, which includes lack of motivation and depression.

The message is clear, to obtain that sustained 'happy factor', and mental energy, it is best to avoid the stimulants that lurk around every corner. Headache medication, for example, often contains caffeine. If you are on prescribed medication you must not discontinue it without your doctor's approval. Over-the-counter medication, however, is often used merely to suppress symptoms, and does not usually deal with the root cause of the problem. By eliminating the bulk of the stimulants discussed in this chapter you may well find that the symptoms for which you are buying medication cease to be a problem. I would expect headaches, migraines, eczema and digestive problems all to be partly or totally resolved by such action.

All stimulants have the effect of causing imbalance in blood sugar levels, and also of triggering adrenaline. Eliminating them entirely is not only difficult for most people, but is also very stressful. It is helpful, therefore, to identify which are the most important to you – which ones do you pale at the idea of living without, and which are your most common 'pick-me-ups'? Some people are better off cutting back slowly, while others prefer to go 'cold-turkey'. You will know which one you are. If you have never kicked your particular habit for a period of time, give it a go. And you could start right now! Resolve that the next two weeks will be a coffee- or alcohol-free zone. You will be amazed at how much better you feel and how much more energy you have.

Here are some good reasons to throw away your crutches, plus ways to help you through the days ahead.

## Sugar

This addictive powder has been nicknamed 'sweet, white and deadly' with good reason. As already mentioned, 80 per cent of the sugar we eat is found in packaged foods, and it is precisely because the food manufacturers understand its addictive qualities that they use it liberally to ensure you buy more. On food lables you will find it variously described as sucrose, dextrose, glucose, maltose and honey. In order for us to process sugar we use up nutrients such as the B-vitamins, vitamin C, magnesium and chromium. Chromium is particularly important for sugar handling, and yet sugar causes a significant loss of this valuable mineral in the urine. You can find chromium in brewer's yeast, wholegrains such as rye and brown rice, shellfish, chicken, eggs, mushrooms, potatoes, liver and fresh fruits and vegetables.

Commercially available sweeteners have found a niche because, although we crave sweet foods, we are also concerned about the downsides of dental caries, racing blood sugar and weight gain. They are promoted to us on the basis that we can have our sweetness and eat it. It is quite difficult these days to buy processed sweet foods which do not contain sweeteners. Not only do the low-sugar and sugar-free products use artificial sweeteners, but so do the 'normal' sugar versions. The reason that artificial sweeteners are incorporated into the normal versions is that they are considerably cheaper than sugar, and this makes their addition very attractive to the food and drink manufacturers – between 0.2–3 pence per litre of soft drink compared with 6 pence per litre for sugar, for example. But artificial sweeteners are chemical compounds that have to be processed and detoxified by the liver, and if taken in any quantity they have the potential to cause significant imbalance in body chemistry, including in the brain. Other types of commercially available sweeteners, such as sorbitol, are made from non-digestible sugars. In small quantities these are not too bad, but in larger amounts they can induce quite severe flatulence, digestive discomfort and diarrhoea.

**Throw away the sugar crutch**
It takes about a month to train yourself to prefer less sweet foods. While we are born with a liking for sweetness, it is only on exposure to highly concentrated forms of sugar that we develop a liking for these foods. If your taste buds have been trained to appreciate sour and bitter tastes, then the assault of

sugary foods can initially seem overwhelming. Gradually cutting down on all sources of highly sweetened foods, over a month, gets you accustomed quite quickly to lower levels of sweetness.

● Cut back on sugar in drinks and desserts, dilute fruit juices with water by 50 per cent and cut back on dried fruit by mixing it with nuts and seeds.

● Check packages for sugar content – some cereals, for example, can consist of up to 50 per cent, making them as sugary as some confectionery. (If you are going to eat candy for breakfast you might as well do it knowingly, and not be duped by the breakfast cereal manufacturers into believing that the sugary cereal is any better.) See **Appendix I** for the sugar content of familiar foods.

● Avoid using artificial sugar substitutes, because while they have no, or little, effect on blood sugar levels, they do nothing to retrain the taste for sweetness, which is the ultimate aim.

● If you get a sweet craving aim to satisfy it by eating fruit. If you get desperate, there are a few wholegrain snack bars which fit the bill, but be aware that many are also very high in sugar. The sugar content will be listed on the packaging, and remember that 25 g of sugar per 100 g (for instance) actually means 25 per cent sugar! Another option is to occasionally spread 100 per cent pure fruit jam thinly on an oatcake or rye cracker.

● To contradict what I have just said, if you absolutely cannot get by without sweetening your food or drinks, use fructose (fruit sugar), but only in moderation. Fructose is around 50 per cent sweeter than sugar and has a small effect on blood sugar. It is readily available from most health food shops.

● Apart from the natural sweetness of fruit, and possibly a

little honey or molasses, there are only (at the moment) two other sources of 'added' sweeteners which seem to have health benefits, rather than detract from health. These are FOS and Stevia.

● FOS (fructo-oligo-saccharides) is a non-digestible sugar found naturally in many fruits and vegetables. While it is sweet, it is also a valuable source of fibre, and thus helps encourage good bowel health by promoting the growth of beneficial bacteria. As it is a fibre, it needs, as does any fibre source, to be added to the diet slowly in order to avoid digestive upset. Build up from 1 teaspoon a day to a maximum of 2 tablespoons a day over the course of four to eight weeks. Once you have done this, it is best to add the powdered FOS by sprinkling it on cereals, desserts and yoghurts. You can also substitute around half of the sugar in baking recipes with FOS.

● Stevia (stevia rebaudiana) is a herb which originally came from Paraguay. Its native name, 'kaa he-e', means sweet herb, and it is quite astounding when you put a leaf on your tongue to find that the intense sweetness lasts for several minutes. Extensive use in Japan since the 1970s, where there is a ban on most artificial sweeteners, has indicated its safety. Liquid stevia is also available, which, as it is heat stable, makes it ideal for sweetening drinks. It is around 200–300 times sweeter than sugar, so only 2–5 drops are needed per cup. You can use it for cooking, but, as it does not have properties which allow cakes and breads to increase in volume, it is not suitable for many recipes.

## Caffeine

Caffeine is such an insidious substance that, if it were to come up for a licence now, I am convinced it would not get approval.

It is so strong a drug that even brief periods of deprivation – of only a few hours beyond the time that caffeine would normally be consumed – can result in significant changes in mood, and symptoms of withdrawal.

Caffeine is not the only problem with coffee. It also contains other members of the methylxanthine group – theobromine and theophylline – which can disturb sleep and cause PMS related breast discomfort and lumpiness. This is why decaffeinated coffee is not always the answer, as these other two chemicals remain.

Tea is now being promoted for its antioxidant health benefits, but it is still a source of stimulants. If you drink really strong tea several times a day you need to consider it in the same light as coffee since, cup for cup, it can provide a similar amount of caffeine. All caffeinated drinks are dehydrating. They cause a net loss of liquid from the body, and so are not really thirst quenchers but instead upset the fine water balance of the body.

### Throw away the caffeine crutch

Coffee is highly addictive, and if you go 'cold turkey' it takes about four days to break the habit. During this time you are quite likely to experience withdrawal symptoms, including headaches or migraines (sometimes quite severe), grogginess and a furry tongue. Remember that strong tea is nearly as bad, and decaffeinated coffee only slightly better. Three or four weak teas daily are not usually a problem.

Once you have managed to stay off coffee for a month, the occasional cappuccino after a meal out will not upset the apple cart too much, but keep it for special occasions, and take care not to slip back into old habits where it becomes a way of lifting energy levels artificially. There are many coffee substitutes available these days, based on barley, chicory and dandelion. While they do not provide the 'kick' that coffee does, they can be an acceptable alternative, particularly if you are the sort of person who likes the ritual of a mid-morning 'coffee' break. Herbal teas are another option, and those that are similar to ordinary tea include caffeine-free Rooibos, or Red Bush, tea, and Luaka tea, which is a naturally low-caffeine tea.

Cocoa is another source of caffeine and theobromine, though, like most things in life, nothing is wrong with a little bit. The problem with most chocolate, however, which is the form in which most people consume cocoa, is that it is mainly sugar (see page 141) and mostly poor quality. The occasional cube or two of organic 70 per cent cocoa solids chocolate, on the other hand, will not do you any harm, though it is quite a strong stimulant. To get a chocolate 'effect' I find the best thing to do is to grate a little on top of fruit puddings – it is so full of flavour that a little goes a long way and can really help to satisfy the urge. Some people find carob bars an acceptable substitute, but many brands tend to be high in unhealthy hydrogenated fats.

## Alcohol

Because sugar is used in the production of alcohol, it has a similar, and sometimes even greater, effect on blood sugar levels. Initially, alcohol inhibits the release of glucose from reserves in the liver, which leads to low blood sugar and thus increased appetite – hence the irresistible urge to nibble with a drink. Alcohol also interferes with the absorption of nutrients, particularly zinc and B-vitamins.

### Throw away the alcohol crutch

Because so many social activities are centred on drinking alcohol, it can feel a little awkward giving it up. The first step is to limit when you have alcohol, for instance never drink on your own at home and don't drink at lunchtime. If you are a regular, but not heavy, drinker (in other words you can set the clock by when you have your tipple in the evening), try the tactic of only drinking on alternate nights. You will find that it is quite possible to go 48 hours to your next drink. You may also find that the effect of the drink that you do eventually have is more intense, as your system has become slightly unused to the alcohol, and that as a result you need less of it. The ideal is to begin with an alcohol-free month, and then to only drink on the odd occasion, for example at a party at the weekend. If you are a heavy drinker and you find it difficult to kick the habit, then you may need to seek counselling.

## Colas

It is not unusual for people to drink a couple of litres of cola, or similar, daily, and to believe that they are not doing themselves any harm. There are, however, several problems associated with these drinks, not least that in drinking them you are denying yourself the benefit of drinking water. Colas are significant sources of caffeine, which makes them particularly unsuitable for young people, who often consume vast quantities of them, and as a result can become hyperactive. They are also laden with sugar (see page 141), one can often containing more than 8 tea-spoons. Sugar-free colas are not much better. They contain such large amounts of sweetener, that it is easy to consume well in excess of the ADI (acceptable daily intake). And these sweeteners have been linked to brain chemical disturbance, testicular atrophy and even cancer.

### Throw away the cola crutch

There are many excellent alternatives to drinking large amounts of cola, including fruit juice mixed 50/50 with sparkling water, sparkling fruit and herbal drinks, such as Aqualibra or Amé, and fruit teas, such as Blackcurrant Bracer, chilled and served with a slice of lemon, a sprig of mint and some ice.

## Cigarettes
. . . . . . . . . . . . . . . . . . . . . . . . . . . . . . . . . . . . .

Everyone knows that cigarettes contain nicotine, but, in addition, every cigarette contains a further 2000 chemicals foreign to the human body, including at least sixteen known cancer promoting chemicals. Nicotine is the main stimulant, and is addictive at even small doses. It only takes, on average, ten cigarettes to get a person hooked, which means that it is more addictive than heroin! And one of its effects is that it acts as a sedative, which is why smokers feel calmer after puffing away.

### Throw away the cigarette crutch
Because it is so highly addictive, smoking can be a hard habit to get rid of. Improved nutrition can aid the transition, however, because it helps ease the blood sugar problems associated with giving up. It may therefore be beneficial for you to first address your diet, stabilising your blood sugar levels for a period of eight weeks, before you finally draw your last lungful of smoke and tar. If you do smoke, remember that each cigarette takes up 25 mg of vitamin C, an important energy nutrient, and you need to replace this. It may also aid your willpower to remember that kissing a smoker is akin to kissing an ashtray! See **Resources** for suggested reading.

## FOOD ADDICTIONS

Certain foods predominate in our diets, and on average 80 per cent of what we eat is made up of only ten types of food. This may seem surprising, but is understandable, when you think about it. The most common foods are wheat and dairy, not least because they are added to many commercial foods as they are cheap 'filler' ingredients. They are also combined in the following typical dishes, many of which you probably eat on a regular basis:

- breakfast cereal with milk
- cheese sandwich
- baked goods such as cakes
- pizza
- pasta with cheese topping
- thick set puddings

With the exception of commercially produced food, there is nothing intrinsically bad about any of these options, so long as they appear on the menu only once in a while. But because they are so prevalent, and are eaten with such frequency – typically we will eat foods containing wheat and dairy products three or four times daily – they can cause problems. This is because, despite the fact that they make up a large proportion of our diet, we are not well adapted to eating large amounts of wheat and dairy products, and as a result they are the main culprits as regards creating food intolerances. Any foods can cause a problem, but the most common, apart from the two I have already mentioned, are the gluten grains (oats, rye and barley), soya foods and citrus fruit (particularly oranges). Symptoms of food intolerance can include bloating, wind, headaches, migraines, eczema, psoriasis, PMS, catarrh and frequent infections. Two of the most debilitating symptoms, however, are fatigue and problems with blood sugar control. The most likely reason these symptoms occur is that when someone eats a food to which they are sensitive, it affects the stress/adrenal hormone response. This is why the foods are so addictive – eating them induces a temporary buzz. At the same time, they may also affect brain chemicals. Food addictions can therefore be every bit as difficult to manage as other stimulants.

### Throw away the food addiction crutch

The main approach is one of substitution, for two reasons. First and foremost it is easier to find alternatives to foods, instead of just doing without. Secondly, if you fail to do this, you run the risk of making your diet too restrictive. Some people find that, in order to make a marked difference in their energy levels, they need to give up the offending food completely, while others find that reducing consumption to more reasonable levels is sufficient.

Not everyone has food intolerances, but many find it extremely difficult to go through an entire day without their favourite food. Around 70 per cent of people who report fatigue and lethargy discover that food intolerances are contributing to the problem, at least in part. But once you get into the habit of having different types of meals, it is really not that difficult. For instance, if you regularly have a cheese sandwich at work you may find that it is just as easy to have a baked potato with tuna or baked beans, or some filling soup and a salad. When experimenting with alternatives, however, it is often the case that you need to persevere. Some foods will be an instant success and you will enjoy them from the start, while others you will need to acquire a taste for. Try different ways of eating them, and you should quickly change your palate. If not, because of growing demand, there is an ever increasing number of foods available which are wheat, gluten or dairy free, and manufacturers are getting better at making them taste the same as the foods they are replacing. All this makes it easier for the consumer to change habits, without really changing habits! Yet be cautious, because the advice to limit packaged foods remains the same. It is also quite easy to become addicted to the new foods, and then you repeat the problem all over again. It is best to rotate and vary your diet as much as possible to avoid this.

The following are substitutes for the two most common food intolerance offenders:

## Dairy Product Alternatives

- soya milk (makes really creamy porridge), soya yoghurt, soya cheese (good grilled as a topping)
- rice milk
- oat milk, oat fibre based yoghurts
- coconut cream (very rich, so dilute by at least half)

## Wheat Product Alternatives

- rye crackers, 100 per cent rye bread, pumpernickel bread (also called German bread), rye flour
- whole oat porridge, oatcakes (check whether they are wheat free), oat flour
- muesli made with variety of grains, excluding wheat
- brown rice, rice pasta, rice cakes, rice flour
- cornflakes (choose a low salt variety), tacos, nachos, corn chips (check whether all of these are wheat free), popcorn, corn pasta, corn flour
- buckwheat noodles, buckwheat flour – make buckwheat pancakes (blinis), freeze, then pop in a toaster when you want one
- millet flakes (to make porridge), millet grains (can be cooked like rice), millet versions of cornflakes
- quinoa can be cooked like rice, also available in 'mixed grain' cereals similar to cornflakes

## FEEL THE FORCE

Man is the only species on this planet that eats foods which are cooked and processed. We are also the only species which regularly suffers from degenerative diseases, and the further we move towards a heavily cooked and processed diet, the worse the array of diseases becomes. Alongside this, we also are suffering from an epidemic of problems related to lack of energy.

In his enlightening book, *Junk Food Monkeys*, Robert Sapolsky describes a tribe of baboons in the Masai Mara who 'fell from their own primordial metabolic grace into something resembling our nutritional decadence' when they learnt to eat food from a rubbish tip brimming with food thrown away by tourists. Their cholesterol went from a level that 'would shame the most ectomorphic triathlete' to levels a third higher, and most of the increase was in the 'bad' LDL cholesterol which builds up plaque in artery walls.

Natural therapists have known for years about the power of raw food and the positive impact it has on our general health and energy levels. Although the beneficial effect it has may seem, to many people, quite indisputable, it is still not fully possible, in scientific terms, to measure its energy value. There is, it seems, something unquantifiable about the 'life force' of raw food. We can measure the nutrients and the calories, but raw foods offer more than this.

Food science is a relatively new field, and it is only in the last seventy years or so that we have identified the majority of the essential vitamins and minerals. Research into this fascinating area of science continues, and thousands of compounds are being identified and linked to health protective features of one sort or another. In the future, these components will protect against infections, arthritis, heart disease, cancer and so on.

Forty years ago, science fiction authors routinely wrote about a time, in the not too distant future, when all we would need for our daily nourishment would be a handful of pills, the tedium of shopping for food, preparing meals and eating being a thing of the past. If some of the giant food manufacturers had their way, processed foods would not be so very far from this science-fiction ideal, and they proudly boast that many foods are now 'fortified with 8 different vitamins and minerals'! (Though they neglect to mention that they are added in because they, and others, have been stripped out during processing.) We will never reach this foodless nirvana, however, because it would lead to significant degeneration in human health (if further decline is possible). There is one key element of food which cannot be bottled, manufactured or synthesised. That is the 'life-force' of food.

Raw foods have their life-force intact. This life force also remains intact if foods are dried at low temperatures or if they are steamed and are eaten when only lightly cooked. The minute foods are cooked at high temperatures, or are heavily processed, they lose their vitality.

Unfortunately, the majority of food eaten, by the majority of people on a typical UK/US diet, is either processed or cooked to the point where all vitality has been lost. You need only look at the shelf space in supermarkets devoted to fresh food, compared with that allocated to processed foods, to get a clear idea of this fact.

Most cooking methods also cause minerals and vitamins to be lost. Boiled vegetables lose many of their minerals to the cooking water, and at the same time the heat destroys some of the vitamins. Cooking at high temperatures also 'denatures' proteins and destroys a proportion of polyunsaturated fats.

On the other hand, we now know that cooking food does liberate some nutrients and that, for instance, a cooked carrot will have more beta-carotene liberated from its cell walls than an uncooked carrot. There is even some suggestion that the reason humans developed such a large brain capacity was that the discovery of cooking allowed more nutrients to be available for the process of enlarging the brain. This may be true, and it may not. The most important brain development may also, it seems, be linked to the types of fats we eat, and that would have nothing to do with cooking. Even if it were true, it is unlikely to mean that ALL the food we eat should be cooked, or that the food that is should be cooked to death. What is more probable is that we need to achieve a balance between cooked and raw foods.

Now ask yourself a simple question. How much of what you eat every day is either raw or lightly cooked? How much vitality, therefore, is in the food that you eat?

As well as vitamins and minerals, proteins, fats, carbohydrates and fibre, food contains enzymes, which are destroyed if they are cooked at high temperatures. These enzymes are probably best described as the 'life-force' of food. When we eat food that still has its enzymes intact, it contributes energy beyond that which can be measured in kilo-calories. How do they contribute energy? One theory is that they spare our own energy reserves, since any food which still has its enzymes intact will be able, partly, to digest itself, saving us the trouble and leaving our 'enzyme reserve' for other tasks.

Raw foods contain a high ratio of potassium to sodium. The correct balance of these two minerals enables cells to more effectively absorb nutrients, excrete toxins, produce energy and regulate nerve transmissions and muscles. In addition, raw food helps maintain the body's acid–alkaline balance, leading to improved metabolic function. Raw vegetables, fruit, grains, nuts, seeds and sprouted beans are also the richest sources of fibre – brans, pectins, lignins, gums and mucilages. Aside from improving digestive function, fibre plays a major part in the efficient production of energy by regulating the transference of carbohydrates into the blood stream as sugar, so helping to keep blood sugar levels constant.

When people are unwell, the first thing they lose is their appetite. This happens for a very good reason. As the body 'tunes up' its immune system for the battle against whatever microbe is causing the problem, digestion shuts down to conserve and redirect energy. Energy is re-routed into healing tissues and producing immune cells. The one type of food that is usually acceptable is some easily digested fruit or a little vegetable juice. We are instinctively aware that what our body needs is food that spares our resources and contributes vital enzymes and nutrients. As digestion uses up around 25 per cent of energy this is a very great energy saving indeed.

## RAW VITALITY FOODS

Including more raw foods in your diet is one of the quickest ways to increase energy. Most people eat no more than 10–15 per cent raw food, well below the 50 per cent required to elicit real health benefits. Eating this amount may sound daunting, but is in fact quite easy to do. To begin with, you should aim to eat a couple of pieces of fresh fruit daily and a small salad as a first course to your main meal. Then increase this to three pieces of fruit, and make sure one light meal, such as breakfast, is totally raw (raw muesli, fruit and juice). If you then add in a snack of fresh raw nuts and seeds, and have a main course salad a few times a week this should bring you up to the 50 per cent mark. Over time you will develop more ideas about how to incorporate raw foods in your diet, and your repertoire will expand.

It is a good idea to build up the amount of raw food slowly, as your digestive tract may not be used to it, and may rebel if too much is added overnight. If you think that raw food accounts for 20 per cent of your diet at the moment, then aim to increase this by 10 per cent every two weeks. In six weeks' time you will be eating a diet which is 50 per cent raw.

**Ways to introduce raw foods into your diet**

● Eat four pieces of fruit daily, as snacks, for desserts or cut up in cereals.

● Use berries and other soft fruit to make delicious sweet sauces for desserts, by just wizzing them up in a blender.

● Make guacomole or salsa for delicious raw dips. (For salsa, use sweet peppers, tomatoes, onion and a little chili, if you wish, and grind coarsely. Dress with a little olive oil and herbs.)

● Eat cruditées at every opportunity for snacks, with dips, or as canapés stuffed with raw dips or other patés.

● Make patés and dips from sprouted lentils, chickpeas and nuts, see **Sprouted Foods**, page 66.

● Freshly made juices are the most delightful way to invigorate your life, and the combinations are only limited by your imagination, see **Liquid Gold**, page 60.

● For snacks favour raw, and very fresh, unsalted seeds and nuts.

● Make raw muesli from a combination of any dried and flaked grains (wheat, rye, oats, buckwheat, rice, millet) and keep in an airtight jar. The night before you are ready to eat it, soak a portion in apple, or other, juice, and add in fresh chopped fruit, dried fruit, coconut and nuts or seeds (pine nuts, linseeds, sesame, pumpkin).

● Salads can be exciting affairs without a limp lettuce leaf in sight. Make a salad with at least ten ingredients: a variety of leaves, a selection of herbs, a large handful of sprouted seeds or grains (see below), any other vegetables, including some you may not have thought about such as sliced fennel, strips of courgettes (use a potato peeler), mangetout, avocado, olives – anything goes. You can also add some fruit, nuts and seeds.

● Soups, such as cucumber, tomato, borscht, can all be made

raw in the blender and then lightly warmed up, but not over heated. The Spanish soup gazpacho is meant to be eaten raw.

● Slowly dried foods count as raw foods, see **Dried Foods**, page 65.

● Sprouted pulses, beans, seeds, grains and nuts can be added to all sorts of dishes, see **Sprouted Foods**, page 66.

● Desserts are a natural for raw food. Ideas include fresh fruit made into ice cream (keep sugar to a minimum), strawberries and other fruit dipped in chocolate, exotic fruit salad. For a tart, finely grind dates, almonds and oatflakes with honey and a little water. Press into a flan dish and fill with blended frozen bananas, raspberries and honey. (To freeze whole bananas, remove the skins, store in a sealed container and then freeze.) Serve with nut cream.

● Nut cream can be made with almonds, cashews or hazelnuts. If you use almonds, blanch them first (pour over boiling water and let them stand for 5 minutes), then pop them out of their skins. Put 1 cup of nuts in a blender with $\frac{1}{2}$ cup of water and blend on high speed, then filter through a fine sieve (if there is too much sediment you need to blend for longer). If you want nut milk instead of nut cream, add more water. Both nut cream and nut milk will keep in the fridge for two days.

Raw food can also mean fish and meat, and there are many recipes for such things as carpaccio, salmon carpaccio, salmon or steak tartare, oysters, sashimi and sushi. There is always a risk, however, of parasites from raw fish and meat, and in these days of mass-produced food it is essential to make sure that your supplier is absolutely first-rate. That said, they are certainly full of all the protein and fat digesting enzymes needed to help spare your own digestive system.

It is also possible to find suppliers of raw milk, although it is not widely distributed. Unlike the pasteurised version, raw milk is much more extensively tolerated and has been used very successfully for various health cures. Again, raw milk comes with its intrinsic enzymes, which help to spare your own digestive system. Bear in mind, however, that raw eggs may be contaminated with salmonella, though, so far, no organic eggs have been infected. Also, raw egg white binds with the B-vitamin biotin, making it unavailable for absorption, so it may be inadvisable to eat too many (for instance in morning shakes or sports protein drinks).

## ANTIOXIDANTS

As their name implies, these powerful substances, found in plant foods, protect us against oxidation, or free radical, damage. Oxidation of our tissues, and of the cholesterol in our blood, has been implicated in the majority of degenerative diseases – heart disease, cancer, diabetes, Alzheimer's disease, cataracts, age-related eye damage, even ageing itself. The potential for oxidation damage is all around us, and is a part of living on planet Earth. Because we are surrounded by oxygen – our most important life giver – we also must pay a price and spend a lot of our reserves fighting off the damage that oxidation can do to us. Visible examples of oxidation occur when iron rusts, cut fruit goes brown and skin gets weathered in the sun. We have enzyme systems in place to fight off a certain amount of this damage, but we are heavily dependent on outside nutritional help to increase our defence against the onslaught.

Fortunately for us, the plant world has the same problem, and they, too, need to protect themselves against the ravages of oxidation damage, especially as it is accelerated by the very thing which gives them their energy supply, the sun. The variety of compounds they use to fight oxidation include carotenes, flavanoids, quercitin, anthocyanidins and polyphenols. There are also the vitamin and mineral antioxidants – vitamins A, C and E, and the minerals selenium and zinc.

Eating a diet rich in a wide variety of antioxidants is the first step to ensuring maximum energy because they support the immune system, help to fight off diseases and spare our own antioxidant-enzyme reserves. Antioxidants are found principally in fruit, vegetables, pulses and herbs, but are also present in tea, virgin olive oil, red wine and chocolate. This is not necessarily a licence to indulge in a 'red wine, strong tea and chocolate diet'. As it happens, you can get the same protective antioxidants from red grape juice as from red wine. The same can be said for caffeine-free teas when compared to the caffeine-laden variety. And chocolate that is made with 70 per cent cocoa solids will contain more antioxidants than the sugar-laden variety. So choose your foods wisely! Ideally, your main sources of antioxidants must come from fruit and vegetables. And because the antioxidants which protect the plants are responsible for their coloration, this means that if you adopt the 'rainbow approach' to eating, and incorporate the following in your diet, you will get maximum benefit:

- a multicoloured fruit salad
- citrus fruit medley (tangerines, grapefruit, red grapefruit, oranges and lime juice)
- grilled yellow, orange, red and green peppers
- rainbow grated salad (raw beetroot, carrot, fennel, cucumber, cabbage and radishes)
- roasted Mediterranean vegetables (put chunks of aubergines, peppers, red onions, courgettes, garlic, tomatoes, black and green olives in a pan with olive oil and roast)
- skewers of multi-coloured vegetables, grilled

- stir-fried vegetables (peppers, bean sprouts, baby corn, water chestnuts, spring onions, cabbage)
- mixed bean salad (mix kidney, chickpea, black eye, butter (lima), sweetcorn, flageolet and soya beans with chopped onion)
- cabbage riot (savoy, red, white, Brussels)

## LIQUID GOLD

If you have never tried juicing, you are in for a lovely surprise. Juicing fruits and vegetables is a great way to obtain a concentrated source of living nutrients – a sort of natural, extra-special, multi-nutrient supplement. And the nutrients are in a form that the body recognises and can use easily, free of the binders and fillers in most supplements. They also have the added benefit of being an absolute pleasure to drink!

As well as being a way of captivating their life force, drinking freshly made fruit and vegetable juices is a highly beneficial way of cleansing the body by eliminating toxins. The fact that juicing and juice fasting is a traditional part of many cultures, and has been for centuries, speaks volumes.

The vitamins, minerals, enzymes and other phyto-nutrients in plants (including those energy-giving nutrients which science has yet to pin-point) are bound in the plant cells and surrounded in a web of fibre. The process of juicing releases the bundles of nutrients stored in this packing, but without the accompanying loss of enzymes that cooking causes. In fact, the nutrients are absorbed directly from the digestive tract without any need for digestion – so we can take advantage of them immediately!

You could, it is true, just eat the whole fruit or vegetable, but the advantage of juicing is that you can have all the energy giving factors of several carrots, and perhaps even a couple of apples, and still have room for breakfast! Generally speaking, you still need to get your minimum daily quota of five servings from intact fruits and vegetables, in order to get their fibre, so juices are in addition to this. But if you know your day is going to be hectic, you can make a large juice in the morning safe in the knowledge that you have had the minimum no matter what the day throws at you.

All you have to do is invest in a juicer, but make sure that it is used and doesn't just gather dust in the corner of the kitchen! Alternatively, you can use a citrus press for oranges, grapefruits and similar, and a blender for soft fruit such as bananas, strawberries and peaches. The best sort of juice, however, is made in a proper juicer which can deal with hard fruit and vegetables such as apples and carrots. They range widely in price; less expensive machines are available from department stores, but if you want something more sophisticated you will need to obtain it from a specialist supplier. See **Resources**, page 148.

So once you have purchased one of your greatest health investments, it is time to use it. All this requires is a selection of fresh, organic fruit and vegetables, possibly some herbs and spices, and some imagination! There are those who say that fruit juices are the cleansers while vegetable juices are the builders and the generators. But really this is splitting hairs, they all contain energy giving ingredients that we can extract and use for ourselves.

Carrots or apples usually form the base, though rules are made to be broken. To this you can add anything you like – pears, oranges, grapes, papaya – or try a vegetable – cabbage is a great digestive tonic that gives a lovely 'green' taste, and raw parsnips are really creamy. Do not be afraid to add bitter-tasting vegetables; as the bases are so sweet this does not come through unless you put in a disproportionate amount. If you cannot afford to go all organic, at least make sure that the bases are made from organic produce.

Some people are strongly of the opinion that vegetables and

fruits (with the exception of the bases of carrots and apples) should not be mixed together, as it may disrupt digestion. I don't believe in making life any harder than it needs to be, and have yet to see any evidence of this being a problem for most people.

If you really want to feel a surge of energy, drink a litre of juice, half in the morning and half in the evening, for two weeks, after which the benefits should really kick in. You can then modify your daily quota to an amount that suits you.

One final word of advice – don't be too organised and juice a week's supply in bulk or freeze it for another occasion. As the living enzymes are destroyed quite soon after being released from the fibre, to get all the benefits, the juice should ideally be drunk immediately.

**Some ideas for juices include**

- carrot, apple and small cube of fresh ginger
- two types of berries in season (cranberries, blackberries, strawberries or raspberries), plus some lemon juice
- pineapple, red grapes, orange and lemon
- pear and watercress
- tomato, celery and fresh basil (the best virgin mary you've ever tasted)
- beetroot, spinach, tomato, red pepper and garlic (with a dash of Worcestershire sauce)
- papaya, mango and coconut
- cucumber, fennel (bulb) and mint (this is slightly diuretic)

## MICRO-ALGAE

Micro-algae, sold in health food shops as spirulina, chlorella and blue-green algae, are the ultimate raw food. These organisms were one of the earliest forms of life on this planet, and as such are at least two billion years old. As a result, they share some of the characteristics of both animal and plant life. During the first billion or so years of Earth's history, the atmosphere consisted of mainly hydrogen, methane, ammonia and carbon dioxide. By using these gases the micro-algae were able to liberate oxygen and so start the process by which the Earth was converted to an oxygen-rich environment able to sustain the type of life that gave birth to mankind. During this time the blue-green algae have remained quietly in the alkaline waters of various regions of the world, virtually unchanged, waiting for us to realise their benefits. They are now being subjected to scrutiny, and one particularly interesting set of trials has shown that spirulina is an effective food source in the treatment of third degree malnutrition. And because of its amazing growth rate, it has been hypothesised that the entire world population of 6 billion could be fed by growing spirulina in an area no bigger than the size of Wales. The Japanese did, in fact, use chlorella during the Second World War to feed millions during times of food scarcity.

Along with other green foods, micro-algae derive their coloration from chlorophyll, the energy factory in plants which turns sunlight into carbohydrates, and which is remarkably similar to the haemoglobin in our red blood cells. Much of the healing properties of these algae has been put down to their high chlorophyll content. Both haemoglobin and chlorophyll consist of a linked series of four chemical rings, although magnesium resides in the centre of the rings in chlorophyll, while iron is to be found in the centre of haemoglobin. Chlorophyll is effective at stimulating the production of red blood cell formation and micro-algae have been used to treat iron deficiency anaemia with impressive results.

Many cultures have used micro-algae in their diets for centuries. Chinese herbalists use them to make up nutrient deficiencies in their patients. The Aztecs of Mexico and the

Mayan Indians ate it freshly harvested, and it was so highly prized by the Aztecs that it was used as a form of currency. Near Lake Chad, in Africa, the Kanembu people eat *dihe*, a cake mixture made from millet, spirulina, herbs, vegetables and spices.

Micro-algae are available in powdered form, and they are also usually enhanced with other 'green' foods such as wheat or barley grass or sea vegetables. One or two teaspoons daily can be mixed in with water or juice, or can be taken directly on the tongue. Spirulina and other green foods, such as chlorella, have been shown to protect against radiation damage and to detoxify toxic chemical out of the body. Chlorella also contains something called CGF (chlorella growth factor), which allows it to replicate at high speed. CGF is rich in RNA and DNA, the very building blocks of life, and it is thought that this may also account for much of its therapeutic value. The protein in spirulina is highly 'bio-available', as much of it comes in the form of biliprotein, which has been partly pre-digested by the spirulina itself. Spirulina and blue-green algae (grown in Lake Kalmath in Oregon) both have an ideal protein balance for human needs, making them a complete food, and although chlorella contains slightly less protein, it is richer in chlorophyll.

These micro-algae are highly effective at alleviating energy crises, depression and mental and physical sluggishness. They can be used effectively to maximise energy levels and to improve mental alertness. They have even been shown to be helpful in the process of withdrawal from highly addictive substances such as cocaine and amphetamines. In fact, blue-green algae is so potent that it needs to be introduced slowly if the person has a frail constitution or is very unwell, as it can cause a 'healing crisis' whereby the person feels considerably worse before they begin to feel better. In this instance it is better to start with spirulina and chlorella and then introduce blue-green algae slowly to the regime.

## DRIED FOODS

Dried foods are not cooked foods. The process of drying, as long as it takes place at a temperature of not more than 110 degrees centigrade, does not reduce the nutrient quality of the food, and retains their 'life force'.

Drying is one of the oldest methods of food preserving and many cultures throughout history have relied heavily on dried foods to see them through the winter or on long migratory trips. With the advent of freezers and processed, packaged foods this art has been almost entirely forgotten, with the exception of dried fruit, grains and beans. Many dried foods can be eaten as they are, while some need to be reconstituted in water. In the case of dried beans they also need to be cooked, or sprouted, as well.

Properly dried food is nutritionally far superior to canned food. You can be sure, if you dry it yourself, that it is free of preservatives and colours, though check that any commercially bought dried food you buy is free of sulphur compounds, the main preservatives used. Properly dried food retains the flavour, smell and colour of the original food, making it very appetising. Dried foods are therefore ideal for meals and snacks on the run, and can be the perfect solution if you need to eat on the go. Busy people need *real* food.

It is easy to buy a dehydrator and, with a little planning, you can create a wealth of dry store-cupboard standbys that will last for several months. It is actually easier to dehydrate than to cook. Usually, all that is required is for you to chop up what you need, or put it in a processor, place it on the trays and switch on the dehydrator for 12–24 hours, depending on what you are making. The preparation can take as little as 5–10 minutes. The result is life-sustaining, nutrient-rich food which tickles the palate as well. It is also a great way of taking advantage of a glut of food, so that you get to eat berries in January without break-ing the bank. If this seems a little daunting, start slowly and treat the process as a different way of cooking. Books and suppliers of dehydrators are listed in **Resources**, page 148.

**Here are some of the possible foods you can create**

- Dried fruits. Fruit can also be used to make more interesting snacks, such as sesame and banana crisps, and cornapple chews
- Fruit 'leathers'. Also dry citrus fruit peel to add to dishes.
- Uncooked whole grain wafers made from dehydrated sprouted grains
- Corn chips
- Plain crackers, using ground sprouted grains, or pizza crackers, adding tomato, garlic, onion, thyme, basil and oregano
- Oatcakes, either savoury or sweet
- Figgy crackers, by adding figs and ginger to sunflower seeds
- Confections using a mixture of fruits, nuts, coconut, grains and honey
- Vegetable soups and stocks made from powdered, dehydrated organic vegetables – dried mushrooms are particularly flavoursome
- Tomatoes (similar to sun dried tomatoes)
- Courgette or cucumber chips
- Dried herbs
- Dried flowers to add to salads (violets and pansies, for instance)
- Fish and meat 'jerky'

## SPROUTED FOODS

Another way to enjoy raw food is to eat sprouted grains, pulses, beans, seeds and nuts. Sprouting is a way of obtaining the nutrients which are stored to make the next generation of the plant – they are pregnant with vitality!

With a little bit of nurturing, some water, air and warmth the seed of any plant can be sprouted with success so that those hard crusted seeds and beans break open to reveal small green shoots. These shoots have big ideas of 'growing up' into strong adult plants. As they need lots of energy to do so, nature has neatly packed these tiny sprouts with an enormous amount of potential energy. The seeds are wealthy in nutrients in their own right, and are good foods to include in any diet, but when they are sprouted they become the millionaires of the plant world.

Virtually all nutrients are increased by sprouting and it is thought that the total increase in nutrient value of sprouting can be as much as 2000 per cent. Protein levels increase by 15–30 per cent, which means they are ideal to add to carbohydrate based meals to make them more balanced. It is vitamins that are the most affected, however. The B vitamin content, for example, increases by 200–1500 per cent, and that of vitamin C by 500 per cent. Vitamin E and betacarotene are also found in particularly good amounts.

The value of grains and beans as mineral sources is also increased substantially. The minerals in plants are often bound by substances called phytates, which makes them difficult to absorb from the digestive tract, but when grains and beans are sprouted the phytates release their grasp on the minerals, making them available to the body. And as if this wasn't enough, sprouts also contain high levels of enzymes and an increased amount of chlorophyll. It is not surprising, therefore, that sprouts are considered to be the most vitally alive and nourishing food we can eat. What is more, they will inevitably be the least expensive item in your shopping basket.

Sprouting has to be one of the easiest forms of food preparation. There is no need to purchase a sprouter or sprouting tray (though they are neater) – a couple of large, clear glass storage jars will do. There are plenty of books on sprouting (see

Resources, page 148), which are inspiring, but below is the basic method of how to sprout lentils. Remember the timing will alter for different legumes, grains and seeds, but in every case you need to use intact beans, seeds, etc, which have had their shells removed – as found in most packets ready for eating or cooking.

1 After discarding any damaged or cracked lentils, place in a jar so that they come no more than $\frac{1}{8}$–$\frac{1}{4}$ of the way up – they will expand greatly.
2 Rinse with fresh water.
3 Cover with fresh water. Cover the top of the jar with muslin or mesh, and secure with an elastic band – they need to breath. Keep out of direct sunlight in a cupboard at room temperature. Leave overnight.
4 Discard the water and rinse. Leave in the cupboard for three days, rinsing twice a day.
5 When the shoots start coming through they can be put in the light.
6 Leave in the light for two or three days, rinsing as before. When they start to go green they are becoming rich in chlorophyll and increasing their nutrient content many fold.

All sprouts will taste sweet and crunchy, and some will taste slightly nutty. You can sprout wheat, rye, oat grains or any other grains, chickpeas, aduki beans, mung beans, in fact any beans, alfalfa (which is the nutritional king of sprouts), sunflower seeds, pumpkin seeds, almonds and other nuts. They can be added to salads, put in sandwiches, and are really good lightly steamed with garlic and other vegetables. They can also be made into delicious dips – hummus, for example, using sprouted chickpeas instead of cooked chickpeas. A handful of sprouts is also excellent as a snack, and if you have a dehydrator you can make a variety of delicious biscuits.

## MENU PLANS

The following menu plans will help you to start on your energy eating plan. They are not meant to be cast in stone, and are intended only as a guide. In changing it to suit your needs, remember the following points.

● The aim is to have a diet consisting of 50 per cent raw food – in order to maximise the 'life force' content. One of the easiest ways to do this is to begin each main meal with a salad, and to finish all meals with fruit. Snacks can centre on raw foods, or juices. You can also make many dishes using raw, sprouted pulses. beans, nuts or seeds – for instance, make hummus with raw sprouted chickpeas. If you are really enthused, making biscuits from raw ingredients in a dehydrator is simplicity itself.

● For blood sugar control it is important to keep snacking. Three snacks daily have been included in these plans. You may find this too much, in which case find your own level, but make healthy, preferably raw, choices.

● Freshly made fruit and vegetable juices do not feature significantly in these plans, although they are one of the quickest ways to boost your energy levels. You can substitute juices once or twice a day for any of the snacks, or have them for breakfast or instead of a salad before your main meal.

Enjoy eating for energy!

| Day | Breakfast | Snack | Lunch |
|---|---|---|---|
| 1 | Rye flakes drizzled with honey, topped with yoghurt and kiwi | Apple and cottage cheese | Hot chickpeas, red onion rings, black olives, shredded crispy lettuce with a thick spicy yoghurt dressing<br>Peach |
| 2 | Citrus fruit juiced with dried ginger<br>Poached egg and wholemeal toast | Sunflower seeds roasted in tamari | Sprouted mung beans, yellow pepper, halved cherry tomatoes and mayonnaise in a hot wholemeal pitta<br>Tangerine |
| 3 | Seeds, fruit (i.e. banana and peach) and oat flakes (soaked in apple juice, if preferred), ground in a food processor, and served in a wide glass | Sprouted beans | Avocado, with apple and cabbage coleslaw with pecan halves and oil and vinegar dressing<br>Oatcakes<br>Plum |
| 4 | Apricot and soya yoghurt sprinkled with raw roasted buckwheat groates | Cucumber sticks dipped in mackerel paté | Marinated tofu and crunchy vegetable kebabs (skewered chunks of mushrooms, cherry tomatoes, cucumber, courgettes, yellow or orange peppers)<br>Strawberries |

| Day | Snack | Evening | Snack |
|-----|-------|---------|-------|
| 1 | Pomegranate | Vegetable juice<br>Chicken, baked red peppers,<br>courgettes and whole garlic cloves<br>Baked potato | Sliced mushroom<br>dipped in<br>hummus |
| 2 | Tahini and carrot<br>sticks | Pineapple ring starter<br>Baked salmon, runner beans and<br>a tomato and basil salad | Corn crisps and<br>guacomole |
| 3 | Cruditées dipped<br>in hummus | Vegetable soup (made from blended<br>raw or lightly steamed vegetables),<br>warmed but not boiled, and<br>thickened with avocado, ground<br>nuts or yoghurt<br>Feta cheese and olive salad made<br>with baby spinach leaves and<br>served with tortilla crisps | Goat's milk<br>yoghurt<br>Fruit |
| 4 | Almond flakes<br>Fruit | Salad Niçoise (salad leaves, green<br>beans, flageolet beans, tuna,<br>tomato, olives, anchovies) | A cup of soya milk<br>and a pear |

| Day | Breakfast | Snack | Lunch |
|-----|-----------|-------|-------|
| 5 | Soaked prunes and Greek yoghurt | Sprouted seeds | Sardines with rye toast and green salad leaves<br>Kiwi |
| 6 | Grapefruit and grilled lean bacon and tomato | Roasted pumpkin seeds<br>Pear | Raw beef tomato, seeded and stuffed with the removed tomato seeds, pistachio nuts, rice, spring onion and basil |
| 7 | Oat flakes and dried apricots with live yoghurt | Cashew nuts<br>Banana | Alfalfa sprouts, thinly sliced fennel, celery and radishes on buckwheat pancakes or warmed oatcakes, served with sheep's yoghurt and mint dressing |
| 8 | Sunflower seed and blackcurrant silken tofu whiz | Brazil nuts<br>Sharon fruit | Smoked salmon 'bits' with mixed green salad and mustard cress<br>Stewed apple with cloves |
| 9 | Small bowl millet porridge served with mashed banana or chopped dried apricots and live yoghurt | Ground sunflower seeds stirred into fresh vegetable juice | Raw beetroot borscht drizzed with mild yoghurt and sprinkled with toasted sunflower seeds<br>Rye toast and seed butter |

| Day Snack | Evening | Snack |
|-----------|---------|-------|
| 5 Pink cheese: raw beetroot cubes in cottage cheese | Bean burgers served with ribbon salad (courgettes, carrots and beetroot shaved into ribbons using a potato peeler) and vinaigrette dressing<br>Nectarine | Tatzikki and vegetable cruditées |
| 6 Mangetout dipped in taramasalata | Turkey casserole with brown rice and lightly steamed broccoli<br>Fruit salad | Hummus and cauliflower cruditées |
| 7 Cubes of leftover turkey mixed with cubes of cucumber | Avocado and leaf salad starter with lemon and oil dressing<br>Spanish omelette<br>Grapes | Goat's milk shake (goat's milk, honey and carob powder) |
| 8 Celery stuffed with organic chicken liver paté | Melon<br>Cauliflower cheese (lightly steamed cauliflower, covered in a white sauce made with feta cheese and soya milk, scattered with chopped pistachio nuts, and grilled) | Vegetable cruditées and taramasalata |
| 9 Pinenuts<br>Pear | Seafood salad platter | Small glass of milk<br>Apple |

| Day | Breakfast | Snack | Lunch |
|-----|-----------|-------|-------|
| 10 | Juiced fruit<br>Boiled egg and rye<br>crackers | Sprouted seeds | Tuna-rice salad (made from tomatoes, pineapple, green pepper, black olives, spring onions and endive leaves, topped with a hot tuna and brown rice mix and sprinkled with parsley) |
| 11 | Sheep's yoghurt and red berries topped with rolled oats | Pecan nuts | Waldorf salad (apple, celery, sultanas, feta cheese, walnuts and vinagrette dressing) |
| 12 | Banana and tofu whiz topped with chopped cashew nuts | Fruit juice and a palmful of roasted almonds | Toasted haloumi or soya cheese and tomato sandwich (on rye toast) with green salad |
| 13 | Buckwheat pancakes with apple sauce and berries | Tamari roasted sunflower seeds | Raw gazpacho with kidney beans and topped with pine nuts<br>Warmed crusty wholemeal roll toast spread with pesto<br>Kiwi fruit |
| 14 | Goat's milk yoghurt whizzed with water melon (include the melon seeds) | Hazelnuts | Curried apple coleslaw on a bed of sprouted beans<br>Rice cakes spread with hummus |

| Day | Snack | Evening | Snack |
|-----|-------|---------|-------|
| 10 | Celery with guacomole dip | Chickpeas and winter vegetable salad with hot spicy tomato sauce | Sheep's yoghurt and chopped dried fig |
| 11 | Goat's cheese and raisins | Spicy parsnip and carrot (juiced vegetables with cumin and fresh coriander) Chicken, tomato and tarragon casserole served with buckwheat | Ground seeds stirred into juiced fruit |
| 12 | Hummus and carrot sticks | Rainbow salad with smoked mackerel chunks Hot baked pear with soya yoghurt | Palmful of trail mix |
| 13 | Sprouted beans | Baked potato stuffed with chopped prawns and tomato, served with mango and watercress salad | Yoghurt and dried pineapple |
| 14 | Raw cashew nuts | Aubergine rings topped with mozzarella and grilled, served with a peach and herb salad with tahini and lemon dressing | Goat's cheese and an apple |

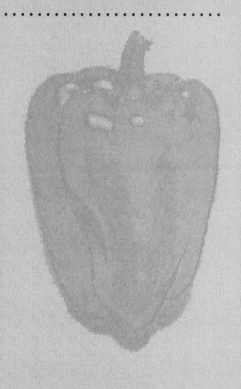

## Part Four

# MORE THAN JUST

# DIET

## THE SLEEP OF THE JUST

Talking about energy can seem a bit hollow if you have just had a wretched night without enough sleep. For maximum vitality during your waking hours it is worth examining if you are getting the best out of your night's sleep. Sleep is not an optional extra to be fitted around other activities, but an essential time for renewal. Some people can manage with as little four or five hours' sleep, while others swear they can't manage without nine, but what is really important is the quality of the sleep. Up to a third of people are estimated to suffer from insomnia and sleep disorders.

It is while we are asleep that our tissues regenerate, and we renew our mental energy. Human growth hormone is only produced when we are asleep, and it is this that initiates the repair of damaged cells. The hormone cortisol, which is normally responsible for breaking down tissues, is at its lowest while we sleep and this also allows our body to renew itself.

Many factors can influence our sleeping patterns, including stress, worry, alcohol intake, blood sugar levels and illness, but it is helpful to consider first the type of sleep problem you have. Is the problem insomnia, where you can't get to sleep; disturbed sleep, where you wake up or are woken up; insufficient sleep, where you need to adjust the time that you go to bed; or do you work shift hours?

Fighting insomnia can lead to its own anxieties and make getting to sleep even more difficult. The following are some of the possible causes of insomnia.

| Problems getting to sleep | Problems maintaining sleep |
|---|---|
| anxiety or tension | depression |
| environmental change | environmental change |
| disruptive environment | sleep apnoea (breathing stops) |
| emotional arousal | low serotonin/melatonin levels |
| pain or discomfort | blood sugar lows |
| caffeine | restless leg syndrome |
| alcohol | pain or discomfort |
| fear of insomnia | drugs |
| phobia of sleep | alcohol |

## WHAT HAPPENS WHEN WE SLEEP?

The pineal gland is a pea-sized gland located at the base of the brain which responds to light hitting our eyes and is involved in our sleep cycle. It produces a hormone called melatonin, and some studies have shown that people who are insomniacs have lower levels of it. Older people also have lower levels of melatonin, and therefore sleep less on average. For sleep to happen, the nervous system needs to quieten. To do this, the level of one hormone, serotonin, is raised, while the level of another, adrenaline, is reduced. Serotonin is converted into melatonin, which is the hormone responsible for regulating our circadian rhythms – the body's natural clock. Melatonin is only made from serotonin during periods of darkness, which explains why people who do shift work, or who fly inter-continentally, can have problems getting to sleep.

### Stages of sleep

A full sleep cycle lasts about 90 minutes and consists of a number of stages.

**stage 1** The transition between sleep and consciousness which lasts about 5 minutes. If wakened, the person will say they have not been asleep.

**stage 2** The first true stage of sleep, still very light, though it is harder to wake the person up. Dream fragments may be experienced.

**stage 3** Moderately deep sleep, which occurs about 20 minutes after first falling asleep. The person is very relaxed and blood pressure and body temperature drop.

**stage 4** Deep sleep. This is the time when sleepwalking or bed-wetting are most likely to happen. After stage 4 we go back through stages 3 and 2 before entering REM (rapid eye movement) sleep.

**REM sleep** All the muscles are deeply relaxed, apart from the eyes, which go through the characteristic rapid movements which give this stage its name. REM sleep lasts at least 10 minutes and 80 per cent of this time is spent dreaming. REM sleep tends to happen more towards morning. People who are deprived of REM sleep become depressed, irritable, aggressive or apathetic.

In the morning it is rising levels of adrenaline, which begin to increase in response to increasing light levels, that wake us up. This releases glucose into the blood stream and gives us energy to start our day.

## SNORING

Snoring can keep you awake, either because it causes you to wake up with a start, or because the noise your partner is making prevents you from going to sleep. Forty one per cent of men and 28 per cent of women snore – in some parts of the USA snoring is legal grounds for divorce! Mucus in the nasal passages is a major contributor to this problem, and the most likely food culprits, which encourage a build up of mucus, are dairy products such as cheese and milk, sugar, alcohol (especially red wine), wheat based foods and soya products. Dust and house mites can also trigger the problem.

It is not always possible to prevent snoring, but natural products, which you spray on to the back of the tongue, and which have the effect of lubricating and tightening the area of the soft palate, can be remarkably effective, see **Resources**, page 148.

## SHIFT WORK

There really is no shift work system that suits the body's natural clock. If you have to sleep during daylight hours you will benefit from fitting total blackout blinds to stop daylight interfering with your body's natural response to light. It is also worth investing in a dawn simulation alarm clock which slowly increases the light level until you are awakened (see **Resources**).

People who are sleep deprived can be prone to inefficiency at work, which in turn can lead to more stress or to accidents and increased susceptibility to illnesses because of a weakened immune system. Junior doctors, for instance, who are on a lot of shift work, tend to be more susceptible to colds and infections than their colleagues who are not.

If you find you are awakened during the night on a regular basis, say by your small child, the best approach is to aim to maintain the four or five hours a night that you are able to get. This anchors your sleep–wake cycle to your body clock. You should then aim to make up the extra three hours or so at other times by napping at the same time each day to keep your body clock in a routine. Napping may help to boost productivity – some of the most prolific people were regular daytime nappers, including Napoleon, John F. Kennedy and Winston Churchill.

## FOODS AFFECT SLEEP

If you are having trouble sleeping, especially if you awaken during the night, one of the first things to consider is whether you are experiencing low blood sugar at that time. A drop in glucose levels in the blood causes the release of the hormones that regulate glucose – adrenaline, glucagon and cortisol. These compounds stimulate the brain, giving it messages to wake up and eat. A light snack of an oatcake, toast, a small bowl of porridge or a milky drink (you can use soya milk) just before bedtime can help allay any blood sugar lows that you might be experiencing in the middle of the night, and thus help avoid the wakefulness that comes as a result. A large meal at night, on the other hand, can have the opposite effect, especially if it causes indigestion.

Avoid stimulants close to bedtime. If your engine is running on overtime it will inevitably be harder to get to sleep. Sugary snacks, caffeine, alcohol and nicotine near to bedtime are all counterproductive. Caffeine, however, is the number one enemy of a good night's sleep as it encourages alertness. When asked to avoid coffee or tea for other health reasons, many people are amazed to find that, for the first time in ages, they sleep through the night. I am amazed that they did not make the connection earlier. Apart from tea and coffee, other sources of caffeine include chocolate, the herb guarana and some pain medication. Other medications, including the Pill, can interrupt sleep patterns, and it may be worth checking with your doctor if you think that medication might be a part of the problem.

A small alcoholic nightcap is not a problem for most people, though a larger amount of alcohol can impair breathing, and cause a shallower level of sleep, as it disturbs the body's 90-minute deep sleep cycle. This can lead to early wakefulness, which is not helped any further by the dehydration that often accompanies alcohol intake.

One way to encourage good sleep is to increase levels of the amino acid tryptophan, which is converted by the body into serotonin. However, tryptophan is not as widely distributed in foods as are other amino acids and, because it is such a large molecule, other amino acids compete for absorption with it (see **Throw Away The Crutches**, page 38, for food sources of tryptophan). Carbohydrates help the uptake of tryptophan by reducing the competition from the other amino acids, but for it to convert successfully into serotonin, vitamin B6 and magnesium are necessary, and alcohol can impair this conversion. Food sources of vitamin B6 include wheatgerm, poultry, meat, liver, egg yolks, tuna, sardines, mackerel, trout, salmon, cod, cantaloupes, cabbages, milk, molasses, leeks and kale. Magnesium is found in all green leafy vegetables, lemons, grapefruits, almonds, seeds, figs, yellow corn, aubergines, raisins, brazil nuts, carrots, mushrooms, crab, tomatoes, garlic, onions, chicken and potatoes.

Melatonin production is enhanced by eating foods high in antioxidants (see **Antioxidants**, page 58). Foods rich in magnesium and vitamins B6 and B3 also help. You can find B3 in wheatgerm, wholewheat, brewer's yeast, figs, dates, avocados, fish, eggs and lean meat.

Eating larger, high protein based meals during the day time, and smaller carbohydrate based meals in the evening can also help because the carbohydrates increase the uptake of tryptophan in the evening. The effects of a large meal at night on the digestive system can also be disruptive since it leads to a rise in core body temperature which can keep you awake.

People on low potassium diets who subsequently take supplements show great improvement in sleeping patterns. To ensure that your diet is potassium rich, eat at least five, and preferably more, portions of fruit and vegetables daily. Sources of potassium are all fruits and vegetables; particularly good sources are potatoes, water melon, bananas and nuts. Colas and similar drinks, alcohol, diuretics, steroids, some heart medication and the herb liquorice can cause you to lose potassium and tip you into deficiency.

Herbal teas such as camomile, peppermint, lemon balm, hops, rose hips, dill and fennel, either used singly or in blends, can help to induce sleep as they have a calming effect.

## SLEEP TIPS

Make sure the basics are right. Is your room well ventilated, or is it too hot or too cold? Is your bed comfortable? Is your bed big enough to accommodate the twisting and turning of your partner – we move 60–70 times each night – or are they keeping you awake? Do you go to bed early enough? This may sound obvious, but people who go to bed after midnight and get up late the next day seem to get little deep sleep.

If you can bear it, get up earlier to increase your exposure to morning light. Sleeping in can reduce the effectiveness of the sleep/wake cycle. On the other hand, low lighting before bedtime helps to have a sedative effect on the pineal gland. Insomniacs can sometimes improve things by keeping the level of lighting at that of candlelight for a few hours before bedtime.

Physical activity helps to ensure a good night's sleep. A busy lifestyle leads to high levels of adrenaline, and exercise helps to normalise these levels, as well as to balance out blood sugar. Higher levels of activity also turn off melatonin production during the day and raise the daytime core body temperature, both of which contribute to enhanced night-time sleep. Exercising in the morning helps to reset the body clock, as does increased exposure to light at this time. Exercise also encourages the production of endorphins, which give a feeling of wellbeing and lead to comfortable sleepiness. On the other hand, physical or mental work, or exercise done after 6pm can increase levels of stress hormones, interfere with the production of serotonin and mela-tonin, and leave you feeling overstimulated. Conversely, relax-ation exercises or meditation at night can have a calming effect.

If your bladder wakes you up, restrict drinks after 7pm, but make sure you still get the necessary two litres of water a day. Older men who find they need to urinate at night may have an enlarged prostate, which should be checked by your doctor.

One study that I particularly enjoyed reading (most of them are so dry!) involved 175 patients of a general medical unit, all of whom were over seventy, who were given a 5-minute back rub, a hot drink of either herbal tea or milk, and a relaxation tape of either classical music or 'nature sounds' to listen to when lying in bed in readiness for sleep. The programme resulted in a reduction in the use of sleeping pills from 54 per cent of the patients to 31 per cent, a remarkable achievement during what, for most of the patients, was short stay.

Finally, reduce time spent in front of computer screens, as exposure to even weak electro-magnetic fields (EMFs) can affect melatonin production.

## SUPPLEMENTS TO AID SLEEP

Various supplemented vitamins, minerals and herbs have been linked to improved sleep patterns, though they only offer symp-tomatic relief, and are no substitute for dealing with the under-lying problems that could be leading to your insomnia. It is of most use to ascertain whether, for example, it is worry, blood sugar problems, or caffeine that is keeping you up at night.

One study likened the action of nicotinamide, a form of vitamin B3, to that of benzodiazepines, the antidepressant and sedative drugs, but without the side effects of drowsiness the next day. One gram daily was shown to prolong sleep time and increase REM (rapid eye movement) sleep. Another member of the B-complex, vitamin B12, has also been shown to help at levels of 3 mg daily. B12 is best absorbed if a sublingual version (liquid drops that you put under the tongue) is used.

The herb valerian root standardised extract (160 mg), when combined with melissa officianalis standardised extract (80 mg), has shown effects comparable to benzodiazepines in a trial with insomniacs. Unlike the pharmacalogical preparation, however, the valerian/melissa preparation did not cause daytime sleepiness and there was no evidence of impaired concentration or physical performance, and, in addition, it does not interact with alcohol. The herb kava kava can reduce anxiety and promote sleep. In studies, 150–200mg of kavalactones taken 30–60 minutes before going to bed has been shown to help people who have trouble in dropping off. Do not take higher doses, however, and do not combine it with other sedative herbs or with antidepressant herbs such as St John's wort. (Herbs must not be taken when pregnant or breastfeeding.)

As already mentioned, the brain chemical serotonin is made from an amino acid, tryptophan, which first has to be converted into 5-HTP (5-hydroxytryptophan). The latter is available as supplements, and has been shown to increase REM sleep by 25 per cent. It also increases the amount of sleep at stages 3 and 4, as well as total sleep time. It is best taken with a carbohydrate, such as fruit juice, to help uptake. The recommended initial dose is 50 mg and this can be increased slowly up to a maximum of 200 mg, though most people find that 100 mg is sufficient. Do not be tempted to exceed the dose, as an excess can have the opposite effect and keep you awake! Another benefit of 5-HTP is that, because it raises serotonin levels, it can help reduce the craving for carbohydrates.

If you suffer from restless leg syndrome it may be worth having your iron ferritin blood levels checked by your doctor, in case they are low, as studies have shown that treating the problem with iron supplementation has excellent results. Do not, however, take iron in excess of the amount found in a multi-vitamin tablet unless you know definitely that you have low levels (for more information see **Anaemia**, page 108). Muscular cramps in the night, or at any other time for that matter, usually respond very well to magnesium supplementation, and you can take 300 mg of magnesium citrate a night. Vitamin E works well alongside this, at 400–800 ius a day (but take only with professional direction if you are on blood thinning medication such as Warfarin). The herb ginkgo biloba may also help, at a dose of 80 mg three times daily, especially if you are over the age of fifty.

In the UK, the hormone melatonin is available on prescription only. Controversially, in other countries such as the US, it is available over the counter, in low doses of around 1–5 mg. The ideal dose varies widely from person to person, depending on their liver function, but it is really only effective as a sleep aid if a person's melatonin levels are already low. A dose of 1–3 mg is sufficient for most people. If taken in excess, melatonin can interfere with hormonal function, and may be responsible for infertility and sexual dysfunction. It has also been linked to problems with the retina in the eye, and with hypothermia (lowered body temperature). For these reasons it is important to proceed with caution when using melatonin supplements in the long term. However, it can be useful for 'once-off' use when going on long plane journeys to help to reset your body clock. It also may have applications for older people with insomnia who generally have lower levels of melatonin. Totally blind people can also be affected by insomnia as they have no perception of light, and their melatonin levels drop accordingly.

Various homoeopathic remedies, such as coffea, nux vomica, arsenicum and lycopodium, can help insomnia, as can aromatherapy, acupuncture and hypnotherapy. There are also a plethora of natural sleep aids available on the shelves of health foods shops, which have varying rates of effectiveness. You may find that if one does not suit you, another will. Their main constituents are usually valerian, hops, passiflora and wild lettuce. Wild lettuce is sometimes called 'poor man's opium', and it is necessary to be wary of psychological addiction. It can also lower blood sugar levels and lead to insomnia in high doses. Hops should be avoided in cases of depression, and valerian used for more than three weeks may induce headaches. None of these induces a hangover effect the next morning, but it is nevertheless best to keep them for occasional use only. Some products contain antihistamines, which make you drowsy, and they should therefore be avoided if you have taken alcohol, or if you intend to drive or operate machinery. They can also produce a psychological addiction, and you may eventually find it hard to sleep without them. Side effects can include drowsiness, nausea and a foggy brain in the morning, but it passes. On balance, the antihistamine types are probably best avoided.

## A SPORTING CHANCE

Most of us are aware of the benefits of regular exercise, but when you have no energy to spare it can seem an effort to even contemplate getting started.

To maximise your energy potential, it is necessary to get into the habit of moving and exercising. You may have heard that energy is neither created or destroyed. But there is one exception to that rule. Energy breeds energy in our cells, and therefore in us. This is because the mitochondria, the energy factories in our cells, replicate themselves whenever there is consistent energy expenditure. They do this to meet the new demand and it starts happening very quickly. After about five days of daily exercise, it begins to get easier because of the increasing number of mitochondria, and you can step up the pace a little. In a nutshell, you are getting fitter.

It is not necessary to change into an aerobics fanatic to become reasonably fit. What is needed is a change in attitude so that everyday tasks are viewed as an opportunity to build fitness. Take the stairs instead of the lift, get off the Underground one stop early and walk the rest of the way to work, cycle instead of using the car. All these measures add up.

We were not designed to sit at a desk all day, travel by car and collapse in front of the TV at night, five days a week. Our ancestors expended huge amounts of energy in just surviving the daily need to find food and shelter. Even our grandparents' generation saw the majority of people working in agriculture and in labour intensive jobs. We have an easier life with many mod-cons, but we are paying a hefty price in health terms. Lack of activity is linked to all the major degenerative diseases – diabetes, cardiovascular disease and many cancers. We need to get moving again.

The average person now walks 55 miles less per year than they did twenty years ago – a drop of 20 per cent from 255 miles a year to 200 miles. And yet walking a mile a day, which takes just 15 minutes at a brisk pace, would enable you to lose about 2.75 kg in a year, and just five flights of stairs daily, for life, significantly lowers the risk of heart disease. So the next time you find yourself circling the car park for five minutes instead of parking further away, think about the benefits of walking the extra distance.

Exercise is vital to improving overall health. The immediate effects may be felt as a stress on the body, but the body quite quickly adapts. We become stronger, with greater endurance, and our whole system functions more efficiently. The main benefits of exercise come about because of improved cardio-

vascular and respiratory function, but ultimately we benefit on
every level.

## The Benefits of Exercise

### Musculoskeletal System
- improves muscle strength
- increases flexibility
- strengthens bones, prevents osteoporosis
- improves posture and physique

### Cardiovascular Health
- strengthens the heart muscle
- lowers blood pressure
- reduces the resting heart rate
- improves oxygen delivery to body tissues
- improves nutrient delivery to body tissues
- widens the arteries to the heart
- lowers overall cholesterol and blood triglycerides
- raises HDLs, the 'good' cholesterol

### Mental Health
- reduces tension and anxiety
- relieves moderate depression
- improves sleep
- helps in the metabolism of stress hormones
- stimulates mental function

### Body Processes
- improves digestion and elimination
- improves immune function
- promotes lean body mass
- improves handling of excess oestrogens
- improves the chances of longevity

Exercise is particularly beneficial for balancing moods and releasing anxiety and tension. It enhances endorphin production in the brain. These are the 'happy' chemicals that exert a similar effect to morphine on the brain, which may be why some people become addicted to exercise!

So if your moods are better, your body is functioning more efficiently, ailments are being kept at bay because of an enhanced immune system, and the energy factories, the mitochondria, are multiplying in number, it is easy to see why exercise, in the long run, enhances our energy levels overall.

## CREATING AN EXERCISE ROUTINE THAT WORKS FOR YOU

The real question for most people is one of motivation, consistency and time. Only about 20 per cent of us exercise regularly. Before embarking on a new exercise regime it is best to consult your doctor, especially if you have cardiovascular problems, existing osteoporosis, muscle or ligament damage, or other serious health concerns. If you are generally healthy, you have everything to gain by introducing a regular exercise routine into your life no matter what your age is. Here are some tips to get you started.

### Pick an activity you enjoy

Finding a sport or exercise routine you really want to do is one of the best ways of ensuring you keep at it. And if you get bored easily it isn't necessary to do the same thing all the time. Whatever activity you do choose, however, it should be of sufficient intensity to increase your heart rate for at least 20 minutes per session, with a 5-minute warm up and 5-minute cool down period just before and just after the higher intensity session. You need to exercise at a level that raises your heart rate, and makes you slightly breathless, but not so much so that you are unable to hold a conversation.

**Here are some exercise ideas**

| | |
|---|---|
| aerobics | skating |
| bicycling | skiing |
| dancing | stair climbing |
| gardening | swimming |
| golf | table tennis |
| gymnastics | tennis |
| heavy housecleaning | treadmill |
| jogging | walking (brisk) |
| rebounding (mini trampolining) | weights (low weights, high no. of |
| sex (remember the 20-minute rule!) | repetitions) |

## Frequency of exercising

To get into good physical condition and to reap the benefits of exercising, you need to do something on a regular basis. It is better to exercise for longer periods of time, at a lower intensity, than it is to exercise for short bursts at higher intensity. The minimum amount to gain cardiovascular benefit is 15–20 minutes of cardiovascular workout (where you get slightly puffed) three times a week. More ideal is probably around 4 hours a week of consistent, brisk movement.

You might vary your routine, for example, go swimming once a week, take a brisk half-hour walk twice a week, play a game of tennis once a week, and do a dance class once a week. By creating a schedule like this it is almost like recreation rather than serious sport, but with many of the benefits of going religiously to the gym five times a week – which for most people would be more arduous.

## Make the time

Sadly, there are only 24 hours in each day. If you start doing a regular exercise routine, you will probably have to ditch something else. The most common mistake that people make is to think that they can just get up half an hour earlier to go swimming or to drive to the gym. The reality is that these initiatives mostly peter out because they do not allow for real life interfering with the new routine. It is therefore important to choose an activity that is geographically near to you, and to pick a convenient time of day. Is it best for you to get it out of the way in the morning before your willpower fails, or is there a time when you usually just watch the television and could instead slot in half an hour of exercise?

## Stay motivated

No matter how committed you are initially to regular exercise there is going to come a time when your enthusiasm flags. Once you stop, however, it is much harder to get started again, so it is better to try and work through such a phase. One of the best ways to stay motivated is to change the activity you are doing, so if you cannot face a brisk walk because the weather is cold and damp, go to the pool instead. To maintain your interest, keep it fun, and make commitments that are difficult to break. If you make an appointment to meet someone at the golf course, for example, you are unlikely to cancel, whereas it is much easier to talk yourself out of a solitary cycle ride. For some people, keeping a record of achievements is a good way of maintaining motivation. By tracking their fitness level, or the number of lengths swum, they get a sense of achievement which spurs them on.

## THE BREATH OF LIFE

Oxygen is the most vital nutrient. Without it we die in about three minutes, and the same cannot be said for any other nutrient. Without oxygen there is no energy. By exercising we increase oxygenation of tissues and improve energy levels. The same happens with deep breathing exercises. Some regimes focus on the two factors together and encourage you to exercise in rhythm with your breathing patterns. Small, controlled movements with focused deep inhaling and exhaling can have benefits beyond the amount of energy seemingly exerted. Disciplines such as yoga, tai chi, pilates and psychocalisthenics (tm) are all good in this way. Aerobic, stamina building exercises such as jogging, swimming, rebounding (mini trampolining), cycling and brisk walking are all highly effective at oxygenating tissues, as they automatically cause you to breath more deeply. If you are upset or under stress, your breathing will change. Breathing is a link between the mind and the body, which we can use as a tool to control our reactions – when you are feeling angry or stressed, you can help relieve some of your emotions by concentrating on deep and regular breathing.

## OXIDATION DAMAGE

It follows that, if we are getting more oxygen to our tissues, there will also be more oxidation damage. It seems odd that the very thing which gives us life, and which is the source of energy, also can harm us, but that's the way it is.

While exercise is needed to improve our overall health it does take a toll, damaging muscle tissue, which then needs to be repaired, and stepping up metabolism, which leads to an increase in oxidation damage. The people who need to be most aware of this are those who are exercising at a high intensity, such as dancers, fitness teachers and athletes. And these people, despite being fitter than the rest of us, are statistically more likely to get colds and other bugs as their immune systems are suppressed by a lot of exercise. But we can all do with a little protection and the best way to deal with oxidation damage is to eat a diet rich in antioxidants – in other words one rich in fruit, vegetables and legumes. Research has also shown that taking antioxidant supplements before exercising dramatically reduces the blood markers for oxidation damage which would normally result from it. The antioxidants used in the studies have been 400–1000 mg vitamin C, 400 ius of vitamin E and 30 mg of beta-carotene. These markers are the result of lipid peroxidation, or damaged structural fats in the membranes of cells. The studies also concluded that trained athletes have an advantage over untrained athletes because their bodies demonstrate improved action of their natural antioxidant enzymes – what the reports do not say is if this is because trained athletes pay more attention to diet than those who are not trained.

A combination of exercise and a diet high in fruits and vegetables helps to improve health because the latter counteracts the very slight negative effect of exercise. Conversely, if you exercise actively and have a poor diet, you will be doing yourself a degree of damage.

## STAY HYDRATED

It is absolutely vital when exercising to stay hydrated. We lose more than 1.5 litres of water daily during normal activity. When we exercise this is accelerated, and it is therefore essential for good health to ensure that the water is replaced. If you wait until you are thirsty it is too late and you are already dehydrated. This will affect your ability to exercise properly, since, when only 3 per cent dehydrated, we lose 10 per cent of the tensile strength in our muscle. One of the best ways of combating exercise induced dehydration is to drink 0.5 litres of water half an hour before your planned exercise, and 0.5 litres just afterwards. You can also sip water during exercise, if you feel the need. Dehydration is also a major contributing factor to fatigue. Coffee, tea and alcohol are all dehydrating, despite being liquids. It is important to drink at least 1.5 litres of *water* daily, and, if you are exercising, to increase this to 2 or 2.5 litres daily. If you really don't want to do this, drink diluted fruit juices, vegetable juices, herb or fruit teas instead.

## BOOST IN A BOTTLE

There are a number of supplements available that can help restore and maintain energy levels. Unfortunately, however, people often expect them to solve their health and energy problems on their own, when this is patently not possible. If a person takes a course of supplements, but continues with an energy depleting diet, there is no way on earth that the vitamins will be anything more than a drop in the ocean. However, if used in conjunction with dietary changes, they can make a significant difference which exceeds that of diet change alone. By making up deficiencies which may have existed, and providing the right environment for healing, great strides can be made.

The following pages list the most effective supplements to combat fatigue.

## NUTRIENTS

**B-complex** Whatever angle different therapists take in treating energy related problems, most would agree that the place to start is in supplementing a good high-potency B-complex. This is because the B vitamins are involved in so many aspects of energy metabolism and brain function. A high-potency B-complex is one that gives 50–100 mg of the different B vitamins.

The use of vitamin B3 alongside chromium in GTF (glucose tolerance factor) to enhance insulin and reduce damage to beta cells in the pancreas is being investigated in trials with diabetics. It may also be useful as a way to avoid the onset of diabetes.

In people with chronic fatigue syndrome (see **Burn Out**, page 125) there seems to be some evidence that their functional use of B vitamins is not as effective as in people who do not have the syndrome. This means that, despite their blood levels of the B vitamins possibly being normal, various B-vitamin dependent enzymes are not functioning as well as they might, and they therefore may need higher amounts of B-vitamins to achieve the same results as normal people would with lower doses.

**Vitamin C** There are many reasons for taking vitamin C, not least because it is involved in energy production, as well as being essential for effective functioning of the immune system. It is involved in carnetine synthesis (another essential ingredient for energy production), is needed for optimal brain function and stress management, and to convert the amino acid tyrosine into the brain chemical dopamine and the stress hormones adrenaline and noradrenaline. It is also a potent remover of pollutants, including heavy metals such as lead and mercury, and thus helps to reduce the body's 'total load'. Take 1–4 grams daily in divided doses. It is best to use a non-acidic version such as magnesium ascorbate, potassium ascorbate or calcium ascorbate.

**Magnesium** This mineral plays an essential role in energy production, as it is needed to make ATP (our cells' energy 'currency'). It also enhances the transport of potassium into cells, which is needed for muscle functioning. Low red blood cell levels of magnesium have been linked in some studies to chronic fatigue syndrome. Magnesium also improves cell membrane responsiveness to insulin, and influences insulin secretion – both of these factors making it very helpful for blood sugar control. Take 300–600 mg daily.

**Chromium** The mineral chromium is one of the main constituents of a substance we produce in our livers called glucose tolerance factor (GTF). The role of GTF is to enhance the effectiveness of insulin. Chromium in the diet comes mainly from wholegrains, rice, yeast and fish, but levels of chromium intake, and soil levels, have been dropping steadily for a while now. Added to this, a diet high in sugary foods causes a net loss of chromium.

As it is quite difficult to get sufficient chromium in the diet, there may be a strong argument for taking supplements. With severe blood sugar imbalance problems it can make quite a difference, as the short-fall in chromium stores are made up over several weeks, so taking 200–500 mcg daily for three months is a worthwhile experiment. The amount you are best taking is weight dependent – the heavier you are the more you need to take. One of the best sources of chromium is from brewer's yeast, but many people who have chronic fatigue problems, or candida, prove to be sensitive to yeast, and they are better off not taking yeast based chromium or B-vitamins. Other successful types to use are chromium GTF, chromium picolinate and chromium polynicotinate. Because chromium is so effective at enhancing the effect of insulin, it is important to be cautious about how you introduce it if you are an insulin dependent diabetic. In this case start at a low dose of 50 mcg, with your doctor's approval, and slowly increase the amount while at the same time monitoring your blood sugar and insulin levels. Your doctor may find that following this approach allows you to reduce your insulin medication over time. For those who are not diabetic, taking chromium may be effective for helping to avoid the condition.

**L-Carnitine** This amino acid is mostly available in complexes aimed at sports people who wish to maximise their performance, but it also has uses as a general tonic as carnitine is used for energy production. We obtain it in the diet from meat (hence its name), poultry and fish, but the body can also make it from two other amino acids, as long as we have enough vitamin C. The people who are most likely to be deficient are vegetarians and vegans. In Europe, carnitine is often prescribed for chronic fatigue syndrome, and for muscle weakness, and this use is backed up by many clinical trials.

**5-HTP** 5-HTP is the abbreviation for 5-hydroxytryptophan, and this unwieldy sounding substance is extracted from the equally unwieldy named plant griffonia simplicifolia. We also make 5-HTP in our bodies from the amino acid tryptophan, which we get from protein foods. We convert tryptophan into the brain chemical serotonin by first converting it into 5-HTP, and this is discussed in more detail in **The Sleep of The Just**, page 79. One of the effects of using 5-HTP supplements is that they normalise serotonin levels, if they are deficient, and in people who experience carbohydrate and stimulant cravings this can impact successfully on reducing those cravings. Doses of 100–200 mg are usually more than sufficient, though it may be best to start at a dose of 50 mg, and increase it over a period of a couple of weeks.

**Coenzyme Q10** This is one of the most widely taken supplements in Japan, with 12 million users – do they know something that we don't? Also called CoQ10 or ubiquinone, this substance is made in the liver, and the raw materials for its manufacture come from the protein found in meat and good quality vegetable sources. We store it in muscles, the richest deposits being found in the heart, liver and kidneys, where it is used in the manufacture of energy. CoQ10 also supports cellular energy manufacture by helping to create ATP (adenosine triphosphate), which is the 'currency' of energy used by all cells. In addition to its energy production function, CoQ10 is also a potent antioxidant, helping to protect cells from damage. Because we manufacture CoQ10 rather than get it principally from the diet, it has mostly been assumed that we have sufficient levels. However, because so many people have compromised liver health, there is a school of thought that CoQ10 is deficient in many people. CoQ10 production also diminishes with age, and if on a poor diet. If you suspect that you have a sluggish liver, you may need to consider whether you have low CoQ10 levels. The main possible symptoms of low CoQ10 levels include tiredness and bleeding gums. Because these symptoms can also be attributed to other causes, especially insufficient vitamin C, it is often the case that CoQ10 is overlooked. Supplements are fairly expensive and levels of less than 100 mg daily are of little use therapeutically. You can, however, take lower doses of 30–50 mg as a maintenance dose. CoQ10 also seems to have important applications as an antioxidant and to help in energy production for people with cardiovascular disease, for athletes and for those with breast cancer.

**Alpha-lipoic acid** ALA is a potent antioxidant that can be used universally throughout the body as it is both water and fat soluble. It is also notable because it serves to enhance the effects of all the other main antioxidants – vitamins A, C and E. In addition, ALA is the only other antioxidant, apart from vitamin C, capable of reversing scurvy. In trials it has also shown itself to be particularly useful at moderating blood sugar levels in those with type II non-insulin-dependent diabetes, and in protecting the body from damage from blood sugar swings. While general doses range from 50–100 mg, levels of around 400 mg are need-ed to improve the situation for diabetics.

## HERBS

The most useful herbs for maintaining energy levels are the adaptogens. Adaptogens are herbs that increase the body's ability to deal with stress, whether it is emotional, physical or dietary. Their effect on the human hormone system has been tested on tangible stresses induced by, say, temperature change, altitude change, shift work or operations. They are not the same as stimulants, such as caffeine pills or guarana, as these not only serve to 'hype' you up but are themselves a cause of stress on the body.

**Ginseng** There are three types, Korean, Siberian and American (though, strictly speaking, Siberian ginseng is not of the same family as the other two). Korean ginseng is the most stimulating, American the most calming, and Siberian lies somewhere between the two. Korean ginseng should not be taken in cases of high blood pressure or breast disease.

**Rhodiola** This is also called arctic root (it grows in Siberia) and was kept secret by the Soviets until relations improved with the West. It has been used by cosmonauts on space missions to reduce the negative impact of space travel on their bodies. As well as being an adaptogen, it also improves the brain's receptiveness to the building blocks of the brain chemical serotonin, making it a useful antidepressant. It is also a powerful antioxidant.

**Liquorice root** Sadly, this is not the type you buy in sweet shops! Liquorice root is a useful adrenal tonic and has cortisol-like effects. Despite this, it has also been shown to counteract some of the side effects of long-term steroid use. It also has useful anti-allergy properties, as it can reduce histamine levels. Liquorice root should not be used in cases of high blood pressure or water retention, as it can cause a loss of potassium, leading to a worsening of symptoms.

**Ashwagandha** This ayurvedic herb, widely used in India, has been shown by numerous studies to be more effective than the more popular Korean ginseng. It has been used successfully in the treatment of chronic fatigue syndrome and can be taken long term for this condition. It also has anti-inflammatory properties which are equal to, or greater than, aspirin.

# Part Five

# TIRED ALL THE TIME

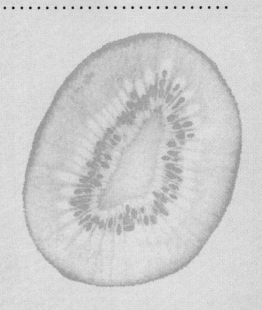

More and more people are visiting their GP complaining that they feel constantly tired. In about 20 per cent of cases tests will reveal a problem such as low thyroid levels or anaemia. But for many people no cause is found and they are told they are suffering from a new syndrome known as TATT – tired all the time. Sometimes their tiredness will be put down to psychological reasons and they will be prescribed antidepressants. However, many patients do not regard themselves as depressed and feel the cause may be physical.

They are probably right. There is a whole set of possible inter-linked reasons why someone may be feeling below par and have flagging energy. In a number of cases there is an identifiable event that seems to trigger the experience of fatigue. Perhaps pregnancy, a bout of glandular fever or a bereavement. But these triggers are not necessarily the underlying cause of the problem. This is just as likely to be a combination of long-term lifestyle, dietary factors and a person's genetic susceptibility. It is unreasonable to expect a test to always reveal these underlying causes. What tests cannot ascertain is the fine balance of an individual's biochemistry. The best way of addressing this syndrome, therefore, is by a multifaceted approach that gives the body layers of energy. When these layers have been stripped away then the result is TATT. But when these layers are added back the result is renewed energy and an enthusiasm for life that comes from such vitality.

With endless physical tiredness, depression, though not necessarily clinical depression, can come hot on its heels. In such cases there are a number of possible tacks to take, and, of course, dealing with the depression is one of them. However, nothing dispels depression faster than feeling physically better, and if you are finding that getting yourself back on an even keel is taking more reserves than you think would be normally appropriate then you can investigate whether there is a physical cause. The easiest to elimate are anaemia and low thyroid problems. Your doctor should also test for a number of other possibilities, such as rheumatism, infections, intestinal parasites or hepatitis. If your test results for these all come back as normal then you may need, depending on your symptoms, to consider SAD (seasonal affective disorder) or CFS (chronic fatigue syndrome).

## ANAEMIA

The most common type of anaemia is caused by deficiency of the essential mineral iron. It is the iron in the haemoglobin of red blood cells which transports oxygen around the body for use by cells. The red colour of blood comes from the iron which, as we know, is reddish/orange when it rusts! If there is insufficient iron, not enough oxygen is delivered to the cells and one of the main signs of this deficiency is fatigue, along with skin pallor. If you complain to your doctor about low energy levels, this is one of the first things he or she should check for by taking a blood test. Other possible signs of iron deficiency anaemia include mouth ulceration, sore tongue, cracking at the corners of the mouth, excessive head hair loss in women, split or brittle nails, which can become flattened, poor appetite, reduced resistance to infections including candida (thrush), poor temperature regulation and poor concentration. Of course, all of these symptoms can easily be attributed to other causes, especially other nutrient deficiencies.

Surveys have shown that the prevalence of anaemia is 4 per cent of the female population of child-bearing age, with a further 10 per cent having a borderline status. This means that one in six women between the ages of 12–55 can be affected by tiredness relating to iron deficiency. Iron deficiency can also have a subtle affect on mental function. Women of child-bearing age are more susceptible to anaemia than other groups because they menstruate and lose blood monthly. In comparison, only around 1 per cent of men are found to be anaemic.

The most useful test for iron deficiency anaemia is serum ferritin, which measures reserves of iron stored in the body. It is more accurate than measuring haemoglobin levels because the level of ferritin, a protein which carries the iron around in the blood, drops before haemoglobin levels do. If the serum ferritin test is not available, then measurements of serum iron and iron binding capacity will give roughly the same information. If you have the latter tests, however, it is necessary to not eat for at least 4 hours beforehand, to avoid a false reading. You also need to avoid having the tests done four days before, and up to the end of, your period.

Heavy menstruation is not the only reason for iron deficiency anaemia. It may also be due to poor diet or the avoidance of certain foods. The most readily absorbable form of iron is haem iron from meat. Vegetarian sources are protein rich foods such as beans, nuts, seeds and eggs, and also fortified breakfast cereals. The iron in these sources is better absorbed if vitamin C is consumed with the meal, in the form of a small glass of orange juice, some fruit or vitamin C rich vegetables such as cabbage or broccoli. While vitamin C improves iron uptake from vegetarian foods, tannin in tea and phytic acid from bran fortified foods, will significantly reduce it. The tannins in a cup of innocent looking tea can reduce iron uptake from a vegetarian meal by two thirds. Recent research examining the effects of a variety of herbal teas also identified peppermint tea as an inhibitor of iron from vegetarian foods. There are also times when our need for iron increases, notably during rapid growth stages of childhood, pregnancy and breastfeeding, and this can exacerbate borderline deficiency. It is also reasonably common for internal bleeding – from ulceration of the lining of the digestive tract, caused by aspirin, steroids, colitis, Crohn's disease, food intolerance or cancer – to be sufficient to lead to anaemia.

Children, men and non-menstruating women need 6.7 mg of iron daily, while menstruating women need 11.4 mg daily. Within this there are obviously individual variations, and women who bleed more heavily will need more iron than those who have light periods. A healthy diet should easily deliver this amount and more. Apart from meat, rich sources of iron are parsley, dried figs, dates, apricots and raisins, beetroot, broccoli, bean sprouts, kidney beans, chickpeas, mung beans, haricot beans, lentils, butter beans, peas, egg yolks, nuts, seeds, coconut, fortified breakfast cereals and shellfish (particularly cockles!). Spinach is also a rich source of iron, though it also contains compounds which limit its absorption. Remember to eat these foods alongside a source of vitamin C for maximum uptake.

If you require supplements to correct anaemia, you will probably have to take them for at least 3–6 months. The side effects of high doses of iron can include blackening of the stools and constipation. You could also experience loosening of the stools, stomach discomfort and nausea. The type of iron that is most likely to lead to these side effects is the one that your doctor will probably prescribe. More gentle forms of iron are available in health food shops, they are also listed in **Resources**, page 148. You may need to experiment with different brands to find one that suits you. If you find that nausea is a problem, take a lower dose and build up, or take it in divided doses. Remember that a small glass of orange juice will double your uptake of iron from supplements, while a cup of tea will cut it by two thirds. It is also worth remembering that iron cannot bind efficiently to the red blood cells if there is a deficiency of vitamin A or good quality polyunsaturated fats. You can find vitamin A in liver, cod-liver oil, egg yolks, full-fat dairy produce and oily fish. As long as we are healthy we also convert beta-carotene (from red/yellow and dark green vegetables and fruits such as carrots, cantaloupes, apricots and leafy green vegetables) into vitamin A, but this conversion is reduced in effectiveness if thyroid levels are low (see below) or you suffer from low blood sugar problems, especially diabetes). Sources of healthy fats include oily fish, fresh nuts and seeds, evening primrose oil and cold pressed flax, walnut, safflower, sesame or sunflower oils.

You may be taking iron in your daily supplement, in which case the dose is likely to be around 10–15 mg. As this is in the range for daily requirements then this is likely to be fine. However, it is not a good idea to self-supplement higher doses of iron unless you have had a test that shows that you are definitely anaemic. The reasons for this are three-fold. Firstly, iron interferes with the absorption of other minerals, especially zinc, and you may find that you are tipping yourself into a different deficiency. Of greater concern, is the likelihood that high iron levels are a significant factor in the development of heart disease and possibly cancer. This is because free-iron, i.e. iron in excess of a person's needs, is a pro-oxidant, meaning that it can cause oxidation damage to tissues. Finally, certain people are too efficient at absorbing iron. This condition is called haemachromatosis, and it affects around 1 per cent of the population. As it runs in families, you should check with your doctor before taking iron supplementation if you have a family member who is affected by this problem.

There are also other types of anaemia. Megoblastic anaemia is where the red blood cells grow very large and cannot divide, due to a deficiency of folic acid and vitamin B12. Those at greatest risk are vegans, people with coeliac or Crohn's disease, those who have parasitic infestations (especially tapeworms), and even users of the Pill. Pernicious anaemia is a type of megoblastic anaemia that results from a deficiency of B12, and prevents the folic acid from doing its job adequately. It is usually corrected with vitamin B12 injections. Other types of anaemia, all of which need to be treated by a doctor, include haemolytic anaemia, hypoplastic anaemia and apoplastic anaemia. Sickle cell anaemia is usually an inherited condition. There is even a type of anaemia called favism, which rights itself when the person stops eating fava (broad) beans, as they lack a particular enzyme needed to process them.

## THYROID

The thyroid controls the rate at which glucose is metabolised and is therefore intimately involved in keeping energy levels constant. The thyroid gland produces thyroxine, the hormone of metabolism. Because thyroxine affects the metabolism of every cell, levels should always be tested for if you are experiencing long-term fatigue. So important is this hormone that every baby is tested for blood levels within a week of birth. A lack of thyroxine leads to a slowing down of all body processes, a lowering of body temperature and sluggish mental processes. The opposite is true if there is an excess of thyroxine – the thermostat is turned up and metabolism is increased, resulting in possible physical and mental hyperactivity. Thyroid disease bad enough to show up in blood tests is very common, and affects 1 per cent of the population a year. You are at increased risk if there is a family member with the problem. When we are under stress sufficient to affect adrenal health, the thyroid can also be affected.

If thyroxine levels are low then the pituitary has to secrete higher levels of TSH (thyroid stimulating hormone), to encourage more thyroxine to be made. Measuring TSH levels is therefore the most sensitive test for thyroid efficiency, and if they are high, and are coupled with lowish levels of thyroxine, then this means that either replacement hormone needs to be considered, or measures taken to improve thyroid function in other ways. If your doctor thinks you need to be prescribed thyroxine, then you should have your levels checked annually to see how you are faring. However, as taking thyroxine can encourage your thyroid gland to further lower production of this hormone, it is generally considered that this is medication for life. One school of thought suggests that it is best to take a dose slightly lower than is needed, to encourage the thyroid gland to continue to perform. There are other reasons for an under-performing thyroid gland, such as an auto-immune problem where the person's immune system is attacking their thyroid gland. Your doctor should also test for these other possibilities. If you are taking thyroxine you need to be wary of high levels of iron (in excess of 10 mg daily), as iron can bind to thyroxine, making it insoluble.

Thyroxine is called T4, and is largely inactive until it is turned into the active form T3. If it is not converting at an adequate rate, then this can be a 'hidden' reason for an apparently underactive thyroid where test results show otherwise. The minerals selenium and zinc are vitally important for this conversion to take place, and correcting deficiencies has been shown in trials to make significant improvements in low thyroid symptoms, including low energy levels. Zinc and selenium dietary levels are commonly below the recommended amounts. You can find zinc in meat, seeds, nuts, wheatgerm, eggs, brewer's yeast, sardines, chicken, carrots, oats, rye, cauliflower, cucumbers, buckwheat, brown rice and tuna. Sources of selenium are wheatgerm and bran, wholegrains, tuna, tomatoes and broccoli, though the richest source is Brazil nuts – just two daily will give a therapeutic amount.

The liver also plays an important part in thyroid function, being instrumental in the conversion of T4s into T3s. As the liver is responsible for around forty metabolic functions, including processing proteins and fats and detoxifying alcohol and other chemicals, a diet that is high in fats, alcohol and caffeine, aswell as being nutrient deficient, will adversely affect thyroid function. If you follow the advice given in the book so far – to reduce stimulants and increase raw fruit and vegetables – liver function should improve dramatically. Liver health also responds particularly well to juices, and to the herbs milk thistle and artichoke.

It is also possible for the thyroid to be sufficiently under-functioning for it to be affecting energy levels, but insufficiently for it to show up on a test. This is a subclinical condition, and it is estimated by some authorities that one in four women, and one in twelve men, are affected in this way. The most likely indication of this is a temperature that runs at below 36.5C/97.8F, when averaged out over a month. The way to conduct this simple test is to take your underarm temperature for 10 minutes first thing in the morning, before you get out of bed (getting up would upset your basal metabolic level). This means that you need to shake down the thermometer the night before and leave it by your bedside – you mustn't even get up to go to the bathroom until you have performed the temperature test. Keep a record of your temperatures for a month and then calculate the average figure. Apart from low body temperature, and tiredness, other symptoms of low thyroid function are puffiness and bloating, especially of the face and extremities, and a coarsening or drying of the skin.

Ways of improving thyroid function centre on providing the

necessary nutrients for building the thyroxine molecule, helping its conversion into the active form and avoiding anything that might interfere with its production. The main foods which are likely to cause a worsening of thyroid function are alcohol, sugar, caffeine and wheat. For ways of easing these out of your life and enjoying other options see **Throw Away The Crutches**, page 38. The three minerals that are most important for thyroid function are iodine, zinc and selenium. Iodine can be found in kelp, seaweed, all seafood, vegetables grown in iodine rich soil and iodised salt.

Certain foods are called goitrogenous, which means that they have been shown to impair thyroid function. These are mainly the brassica family of broccoli, cabbage, Brussels sprouts and cauliflower. These are, however, extremely good foods in many respects, and are cancer-preventative, so it is not a good idea to avoid them totally, especially as it is only in significant amounts – a large portion daily – that they exert their effect. However, if you have low thyroid function, limiting them to three or four times a week may be a good policy, but make sure that you substitute other green leafy vegetables, such as leeks and spinach, instead. Another food that may interfere slightly with thyroid function, but which is generally regarded as a healthy option, and cancer protective, is soya, and it may also be prudent to restrict consumption of this to three or four times a week if you have a low thyroid output.

Supplements can help to normalise thyroid function, though it is necessary to work on the diet first. Spirulina has had a substance called thyroxine factor isolated by Russian scientists, which may nourish the thyroid and help to normalise metabolism (see **Micro-algae**, page 62). Kelp is one of the most popular supplements as it is a rich source of iodine as well as other trace minerals. Kelp has been shown to prevent goitre – a swelling of the thyroid gland, leading to a thick, bulbous neck, and the sign of a very underactive thyroid. Kelp should not be taken by people with overactive thyroids as it may speed up thyroid function by giving them too much iodine, and it can even lead to goitre if taken in excessive amounts. Large doses of iodine, for instance from iodised salt, may cause an increase in thyroid hormone release, due to an overactive thyroid (hyperthyroidism) or a drop in thyroid hormone (hypothyroidism). A dose of 100 mcg daily should be sufficient for most people. There are a number of specialised thyroid-supporting supplements which combine the amino acid tyrosine, which makes up part of the thyroxine molecule, with iodine and other supporting herbs. Some of these are listed in **Resources**, page 148.

Filter your water, as chemicals and waste products which accumulate in our water, including phthalate esters from plastic water bottles and chlorine from tapwater, have been shown in several studies to lower levels of thyroid hormones. Fluoride can also suppress thyroid function and a priority is to ensure that your drinking water is fluoride free. Numerous people with suppressed thyroid glands have returned to normal after eliminating fluoride.

## SAD IN THE WINTER?

If your energy levels are significantly lower in the winter months it is always possible that you are experiencing SAD (seasonal affective disorder). SAD can be distinguished from other illnesses, such as chronic fatigue, because its symptoms are only present on a seasonal basis, and disappear completely in spring and summer. It is estimated that around 5 per cent of people who live in countries in the northern hemisphere are affected by SAD, though many more than this may complain of feeling 'out of sorts' in the winter months. (In countries which are below the equator few incidences of SAD are found.) Undoubtedly, as with most other health problems, there are variations, and many people have a subclinical version of SAD.

There are four classic, major, symptoms experienced in the autumn and winter by most people who suffer from SAD and these are:

- increased desire to sleep
- extreme lethargy
- depression
- increased appetite, often leading to weight gain

There are many other possible symptoms which are exacerbated in the winter and which some, but not all, SAD sufferers might encounter:

- an inability to cope with stress
- phobias
- avoidance of social situations
- loss of libido
- sleep disturbance
- mood swings
- premenstrual tension
- comfort eating
- increased headaches, muscle or joint pains
- digestive disturbances
- palpitations

Those affected may find that, despite the fact that they do less in the winter, they still feel tired and want to sleep more, but their sleep is often restless and unrefreshing. They may also find that they are unmotivated and unable to concentrate at work. Many SAD sufferers will put on an average of 4 kg in the winter, probably as a result of eating more in an effort to replenish energy stores, and will behave almost like an animal going into hibernation. Depression is a major symptom of SAD, and low self-esteem, guilt, hopelessness, anxiety and despair weigh down many sufferers. There are, however, significant differences between people with SAD and those with classical depression.

| Classical depression | SAD |
| --- | --- |
| no seasonal pattern | repeated seasonal pattern |
| difficulty sleeping | a need to sleep more |
| loss of appetite | a need to eat more |
| loss of weight/stable weight | increase in weight |
| mood not influenced by number of daylight hours | mood influenced by number of daylight hours |

The return to full health in the spring and summer months is welcome, however the transition phase is not always without problems. In most cases the return to normal energy levels is simply a divesting of the torpor of the winter months. But in some cases 'spring mania' is experienced. This hypomania can be a sense of elation, accompanied by a degree of hyperactivity, which can irritate all around them. It may involve talking or acting irrationally, being distracted, sleeplessness, a need to seek greater excitement out of life, financial extravagance and differing perceptions to people around them.

## IS LIGHT THE FORGOTTEN NUTRIENT?

As we learn more about the effects of light on the human body, more questions must be raised about the impact of spending large amounts of time in buildings with high levels of substandard artificial lighting. We are more aware of the effects of light on plants and animals than we are on humans. Plants without light cannot survive, as they cannot synthesise food, and animals are influenced by light in their migratory and hibernation patterns. Light is taken in through the eye, and affects the pineal gland, which in turn exerts a regulating effect on the hormone systems of the body. Natural light also triggers melanin (as opposed to melatonin) in the skin, and synthesises vitamin D in our skin for use by the whole body.

The light that fulfils all of these functions is full spectrum light, which includes ultra violet rays that can penetrate the skin to trigger production of vitamin D. If it can do this, then it is of sufficient intensity to regulate the hormonal mechanisms. Most indoor lighting is unable to do this. One of the main treatments for SAD is the use of full spectrum light boxes, which leads to improvement in 70–80 per cent of SAD sufferers. It seems that the antidepressant effect of light boxes is most effective if they are used in the morning, however there are many different regimes and types of light boxes, and it is best to get specialist information. Some studies have also shown that the effectiveness of light boxes is enhanced if high-density, negative ion treatment is used alongside. These are boxes which change the electrical charge of the air to more closely approximate the type of ions found in air near the sea, rather than those found in air in inner cities.

As already mentioned in **The Sleep of The Just**, melatonin is the hormone responsible for setting our body clocks. Research seems to indicate that people with SAD have levels of melatonin that alter several hours earlier than in normal people, and this is true for both the evening rise in levels and the morning decline. This suggests that their biological clocks may be delayed or running slow. It is now thought that people with SAD have deficiencies in certain brain chemicals, particularly serotonin and dopamine. This would accord with many of the symptoms of SAD, as, for instance, low serotonin levels are linked to carbohydrate cravings and depression. Studies have also shown that drugs which stimulate serotonin production have been fairly successful at treating SAD. Logic therefore dictates that supplements, such as 5HTP and the herb rhodiola, which help to increase serotonin levels, should also benefit those with SAD.

Another important aspect of sun exposure is that it is needed to manufacture vitamin D in the skin, which is essential for correct metabolism of calcium for bone health. Children who receive low levels of sun exposure, either because they are dark skinned and have a dress code which dictates that they cover up almost totally, or because they are bedridden and unable to go out, can have such severe vitamin D deficiency that rickets results. More commonly, low levels of vitamin D in sun-starved adults has been linked to osteomalacia, osteoporosis and hormonal diseases such as breast and prostate cancers. A fair-skinned person can generate sufficient vitamin D for the day's needs in half an hour of sun exposure in the spring or summer. This is not the same as being locked indoors on a daily basis and then getting the majority of sun in a two-week block on holiday. It is not possible to make up deficiency in this way, and of course it is harmful to expose yourself to the sun at high intensity.

## EATING TO COMBAT SAD

SAD sufferers tend to eat more in the winter months and their food preferences can also change. Much of the increased eating is aimed at gaining relief from symptoms such as anxiety or fatigue. Carbohydrate cravings for starchy or sugary foods seems to be the worst problem. It is also common to turn to stimulants such as coffee, alcohol, sugar and chocolate. Interestingly, however, not all SAD sufferers crave carbohydrates, some will turn to high protein foods. Understanding which foods affect your moods is a powerful way of reducing the impact of SAD.

The first step is to understand your reactions to the two main food groups just mentioned – proteins and carbohydrates – because these are the foods which govern the balance of serotonin, noradrenaline and dopamine. To do this, chose a week when you can concentrate on your eating habits and note how your mood is affected. Stock up on a selection of foods which you enjoy to eat in the coming week. There should be enough proteins to form the basis of seven days' worth of protein meals: meat, fish, eggs, cheese, milk, yoghurt, cream, tofu, lentils, beans. There should also be enough carbohydrates for seven days' worth of carbohydrate meals: pasta, potato, rice, bread, oats, rye, buckwheat, root vegetables, bananas, watermelon, grapes, sugars. You can also use skimmed milk with carbohydrate meals. The object of the exercise is not to eat an optimal diet (for example, sugar and cream have been listed), but to find out the effect of food on the way you experience SAD. Of course, if you are already avoiding certain foods then continue to do so! Each type of meal can be accompanied by cooked or raw vegetables or topped with vegetable sauces. You can also use fats such as oils or butter with either type of meal. You will need, too, to stock up on suitable snacks – ideally low-sugar fruit not mentioned above (i.e. oranges, apples, strawberries, etc). You should avoid alcohol entirely, and ideally coffee and tea too, though if you have not already stopped using them then carry on at a low level of three weak cups daily, as abruptly stopping them may interfere with your moods.

You now need a notebook to record what you eat, when you eat, and in what way you are affected by your food choices. You need to alternate between pure protein meals and pure carbohydrate meals as follows:

**DAY 1**   carbohydrate breakfast
protein lunch
carbohydrate evening meal

**DAY 2**   protein breakfast
carbohydrate lunch
protein evening meal

For Days 3–7 alternate between Day 1 and Day 2.

How much you eat at each meal is not important, but it is essential that you do not mix proteins with carbohydrates. Here are some ideas for different types of meals:

## carbohydrate breakfasts
- fruit juice
- toast with butter and jam or honey (avoid nut butters)
- muesli or other cereal with skimmed milk or banana
- porridge with skimmed milk and honey

## protein breakfasts
- eggs with mushrooms (no toast)
- smoked fish (i.e. kipper or mackerel) with tomato
- low fat yoghurt with low-sugar fruit
- cottage cheese with low-sugar fruit
- thick breakfast shake made with unsweetened soya milk, 50 g silken tofu, and soft fruit such as strawberries and peaches (not banana)

## carbohydrate main meals
- baked potato with butter or sour cream and salad
- pasta with tomato, mushroom, olive, onion, garlic or herb based sauce

- rice with stir fried vegetables, or with vegetable curry
- wholemeal sandwich or pitta pocket made with avocado, tomato, onion, cucumber, sprouts and lettuce
- main course salad with a variety of vegetables and new potatoes or pasta shapes
- thick vegetable soup with rice or pasta shapes

**dessert**
- cake, biscuit, chocolate

**protein main meals**
- fish – baked, steamed, poached or canned – served with vegetables
- grilled meat or chicken, served with vegetables
- meat, chicken or fish based casserole using lots of vegetables but no potatoes, rice or bread
- eggs – i.e. mushroom and leek omelette, herb, garlic, onion and Parmesan omelette, tomato and grated courgette omelette (no potatoes or bread)
- cheese with vegetables – i.e. celery with cream cheese sprinkled with paprika, three coloured peppers with cottage cheese, or Mediterranean vegetables with grilled goat's cheese
- tofu – i.e. stir fried marinated tofu, tofu kebab, vegetarian shepherd's pie with tofu mashed up in to it
- large salad with many vegetables and topped with fish, meat or cheese of choice, or tofu

**dessert**
- plain natural yoghurt or a little cheese

These meals are not meant to be nutritionally exemplary (hence the biscuits and cake for dessert with the carbohydrate meal).

What they are intended to do is to segregate the different types of foods as they might affect your moods. After a meal, allow 2 hours to go by before you snack, and then have either a protein or a carbohydrate snack, or fruit.

After each meal or snack you need to evaluate how you are feeling. The following are some possible words and phrases to use to describe this, though you may have others you think more appropriate!

- alert, calm, refreshed, relaxed, energetic, enthusiastic, able to concentrate
- lethargic, tired, 'woolly' brained, anxious, depressed, agitated, tearful

You can also note any particular cravings that you may have had.

At the end of the week you should be able to look back and assess the impact that diet is having on your moods. Did you notice any change before and after eating particular types of meals? Did you crave particular foods? Did protein meals or carbohydrate meals give you more energy, stimulate you more or give you the ability to concentrate better?

For optimal health we need a balance of different types of food, however you may find that you are now able to time the types of meals you have to influence your moods to best effect. For instance, if you find that protein meals invigorate you, whereas carbohydrates have the opposite effect, then your breakfasts and lunches should consist of protein based choices, leaving you to enjoy your carbohydrate meals in the evening to help you sleep and relax. If, on the other hand, you find that carbohydrate meals energise you then your eating pattern should be the other way round.

You can also get a good sense of what is the best timing for you for various meals and snacks. If you find that you crave a sugar snack around 4 or 5 pm, then just before this, say around 3.30 pm, is the time to have a more appropriate slow-releasing carbohydrate snack to energise instead of deflate you. Having said earlier that quantity did not matter for the week-long experiment, remember that in the long run heavy, fatty meals will be harder to digest and that eating more frequent, lighter meals may help to keep your energy levels constant.

Incorporating lots of fruit and vegetables is also one of the best ways to optimise your energy levels if you are affected by SAD. While sunlight is the most important factor for boosting levels of melatonin, a diet rich in antioxidants helps to boost melatonin levels as well. Antioxidant rich foods to increase your intake include:

- all fruit and vegetables, and in particular the red/purple/yellow/orange coloured ones
- legumes, particularly soya beans
- dark green extra virgin olive oil
- teas such as Japanese green tea, South African red bush tea, rosehip tea and black teas (but remember to drink weak tea because of its high caffeine content)

## BURN OUT

Variously called CFS (chronic fatigue syndrome), ME (myalgic encephalomyelitis), post viral fatigue syndrome, adrenal syndrome, and even yuppie flu, this is the ailment that dare not speak its name, and it has only been recognised as a true ailment in the last decade. It affects an estimated 100,000 people in the UK, 70 per cent of whom are women, and is probably most accurately described as CFS, because there appear to be a number of contributing factors. These may include a poor recovery from viral infection, or impaired adrenal function, but not necessarily.

There is not even a consensus on what it is or how to diagnose it, though doctors now have a check list of possible factors which lead to a diagnosis and there is a reasonable chance that someone afflicted by CFS will not be dismissed as a hypochondriac or a work-shy malingerer. Increasingly, there is awareness amongst doctors that it is unhelpful to try to make distinctions between the physical and mental arenas when treating this problem, and that the contributing factors are likely to be very individual. There are no reliable tests for CFS, though ones are being developed based on the fact that many people with CFS seem to have reduced levels of the brain chemical serotonin.

The main manifestation is an inexplicable burn out, sufficiently serious to hamper participation in most daily activities. One reason why women are more likely to be affected may be because of an imbalance of female hormones throughout the menstrual cycle. The fatigue can be accompanied by aches and pains, disturbed vision, low grade fever, an inability to concentrate ('woolly brain syndrome'), reduced appetite and an inability to cope with any physical or mental stress. One person, when asked to describe their symptoms, said 'Imagine you have just finished running a marathon, have a migraine headache and a bad attack of flu – that is how I feel all the time!'. The worst affected can suffer severe pain and short-term memory loss, and be unable to walk even short distances – in the worst cases they can be bedridden. I have also known people who needed to spend several hours recovering after having crawled up the stairs on their hands and knees. For most sufferers the daily battle is one of maintaining a semblance of normality while they aim to overcome the restrictions imposed on them by their condition.

## Criteria for Chronic Fatigue Syndrome

1  Fatigue lasting for at least six months.
2  Fatigue which is made worse by physical or mental exertion, lasts for a significant amount of time and is not relieved by rest.
3  Painful lymph nodes in the neck, sore throat, mild fever or chills.
4  Unexplained muscle weakness, muscle pain (myalgia), joint pain without swelling.
5  Short-term memory problems, forgetfulness, inability to concentrate, 'woolly' head, headaches, nausea.
6  Digestive problems.
7  Depression (but not necessarily clinical depression).
8  Sleep disturbance.

These symptoms have to persist for at least six months in order to comply with the definition of CFS, though you do not have to suffer from all of them. Most of the symptoms characteristic of CFS could also be caused by other chronic diseases, such as hypothyroidism, rheumatoid arthritis, eating disorders, substance abuse or cancer, and it is necessary to rule out other possible contributing factors first.

It is common for those with CFS to have had a bout of serious viral disease in the past, such as Epstein Barr (glandular fever or mononucleosis) or coxsackie (a group of enteroviruses, or gut bugs, linked to aseptic meningitis). These diseases obviously do not affect everyone in the same way, as 90 per cent of people have Epstein Barr antibodies in their blood by the age of thirty, indicating that they have been in contact with the virus. It remains latent in the body but may become active and create typical glandular fever symptoms if the immune system is unable to keep the virus in its dormant state. The first mistake often made by those with CFS is to return to work after having had one of these viruses whilst they are still weak from the illness, leading to what is best called post-viral syndrome. This can co-exist with under-functioning adrenal glands. If the person has an inherited tendency to low adrenal function, or if the adrenal glands are chronically overtaxed, they are not up to the job of coping when under stress, or when recovering from illness. This is called functional depletion, and it is distinct from the physical atrophy of the adrenal glands that occurs in Addison's disease. CFS is probably best thought of as a provocation disease. In other words, a range of factors – a virus, bacterial infection, stress, surgery, vaccination, an allergic tendency, toxic chemicals – can accumulate, causing a susceptible person to succumb. In one study, 80 per cent of biopsies showed evidence of damage to the mitochondria, the energy factories in cells.

Resolving CFS can take quite a long time – in some cases years. It is important to acknowledge this, otherwise overtaxing yourself at times when you are feeling better can lead to a relapse, which in turn can lead to depression. It is also advisable to take a multi-faceted approach that encompasses several disciplines, and the best results seem to be achieved by using a combination of diet, nutritional supplements, stress management or counselling, homoeopathy, acupuncture and physiotherapy. A highly successful trial at Glasgow Homoeopathic Hospital recorded improvements in 70 per cent of CFS patients when they followed a wheat-free diet, used nutritional supplements, were screened for allergies, avoided fluoride, took homoeopathic remedies and had physiotherapy treatment.

It is also advisable to get the help of a qualified nutritionist, who can speed recovery by running tests to reveal what specific nutrient deficiencies may be involved. The best nutritional strategy is one that supports the body's whole adaptive mechanism (see Hans Selyé, page 23), and includes enhancing the immune system's ability to cope with the various 'loads' that are placed upon it, whilst simultaneously reducing those loads – for instance, pollution, toxins, candida, allergies and food intolerances. The most important nutritional tools for dealing with CFS are as follows.

**Eat a nutrient-dense diet** A healthy, preferably organic, diet is essential to maximise energy levels and promote recovery. Eat plenty of high energy foods such as fruit, vegetables, lentils, pulses, brown rice, oats, barley and fresh fish. Favour oils which are healthy, and ideally cold-pressed, such as extra virgin olive oil, linseed and walnut oils. Completely avoid hydrogenated fats – found in margarines, and in packaged foods such as crisps, biscuits and pies (including vegetarian foods). Eat to balance blood sugar levels and make sure that you eat five small meals and snacks daily. By avoiding large meals you will conserve energy. It is also strongly advisable to avoid all sources of caffeine and alcohol. If you are already drinking these, then reduce them gradually over a couple of weeks to avoid a rebound reaction and headaches. Drink 2 litres of water daily for hydration and cleansing of your body tissues and organs. Keep sources of sweetness to fruits, a little honey, a little fructose, FOS or stevia. Irrespective of whether you have candida or not (see below), sprinkle cracked linseeds or psyllium husks on your cereals or in drinks daily, to improve digestive function and aid the elimination of toxins from the body.

**Food sensitivities** These can be a particular problem for people with CFS, and in general it is certainly best to follow a wheat free diet, and possibly also to investigate other sensitivities, especially to dairy produce. Follow the advice in **Throw Away The Crutches**, page 38. The information regarding stimulants is particularly relevant to those with CFS.

**Dietary salt** The typical person eats far too much salt – around 9 grams daily, compared with the recommended 6 grams – and the majority of this, around 80 per cent, comes from packaged foods. Generally speaking, most people will benefit from reducing the amount of salt in their diet, as it can help lower high blood pressure and reduce the risk of cardiovascular problems. However, one fairly constant finding in those with CFS is that they have what is called postural hypotension. This is low blood pressure, particularly when the body goes from a lying position to a standing one. When challenged in this way the body's stress mechanisms are unable to respond and make the transition a smooth one. There is some evidence that increasing salt levels in the diet helps to maintain more normal blood pressure and relieves some of the effects associated with postural hypotension, such as feeling faint. However, this is only true of people who have been on a prolonged salt restricted diet, in which case they may want to experiment with increasing their salt intake to the maximum recommended amount of 6 grams daily.

**Candida** This is an overgrowth of an opportunistic yeast organism. The most common candida is candida albicans, and it is normally resident in the bowels. It is, however, a highly opportunistic organism and, if the immune system of a person is weakened, there is a greater chance of it growing in other areas. Most commonly, this manifests as thrush, which leads to a white discharge and itchiness in the vagina or anal area. Thrush of the mouth, eyes, under the nails or other areas is also quite common. Occasionally, however, the candida manages to invade higher up the digestive tract, in the small intestines, and affects other body tissues. In such cases the person can feel quite debilitated, with lack of energy being one of the most severe problems. There are often a host of other related problems, too, such as food allergies, sensitivities to moulds and damp environments, headaches and migraines. It was particularly common, at one point, for all people with CFS to be diagnosed with candida. This probably came about because the medical profession did not acknowledge CFS, and have also been cautious about recognising candida. This meant that other therapists would often lump the two together because the symptoms can often seem to mirror each other. We now know that although it is likely that candida is present in a significant number of cases of CFS, around 25 per cent, CFS is quite a different condition.

Treating candida, if it is present, is one of the most important aspects of dealing with CFS. However, it is important that it is handled properly, for two reasons. Firstly, if the person goes on too restricted a diet, then this can be detrimental to recovery from CFS, and, secondly, if the candida is treated too aggressively then this can result in 'die-off'. Die-off is where the dead yeast, which has not managed to thrive because dietary and supplement treatments have made the environment too hostile for it to survive, is more toxic (in the short term) than the candida itself. The person can find that a reaction to die-off is very debilitating, and this can be worse if the person has CFS.

The main dietary advice for getting rid of candida is to rigorously avoid all sources of sugar because the yeast feeds on it – as it does in familiar processes such as bread making and brewing. In addition to cutting out sugar, sugar containing products, fast-releasing carbohydrates which turn into sugar quite speedily and alcohol, it may also be necessary to cut back on over-ripe fruit and instead stick to fruit such as green apples and pears. Most of the measures already described in this book will be appropriate for an anti-candida diet. The other main dietary treatment is to avoid all yeasts – in the form of bread (apart from unleavened varieties, such as soda bread and oatcakes), alcohol (again), most cheeses (though cottage cheese is OK), Quorn, vinegars and, in extreme cases, mushrooms. It is also necessary to avoid stimulants and any foods to which you may be sensitive or allergic.

It is necessary, too, to improve bowel health by taking some gentle fibre to help the body eliminate the yeast organisms. The best way to do this is to take either two tablespoons of cracked linseeds daily (add to cereals or yoghurts), or two teaspoons of psyllium husks (add to juice and drink down quickly). If you are unused to a diet high in fibre, begin with less and build up slowly to the full dose. And make sure you drink a large glass of water after taking either of these fibres, to allow them to swell in the digestive tract. It is also helpful to take a 'probiotic' supplement that includes lactobacillus acidophilus and bifidobacteria. Probiotics are healthy bacteria (the opposite of antibiotics), and are needed in the bowels to fill in the spaces left behind by the killed off candida.

In addition to these treatment options, there are also a number of anti-candida supplements, as well as over-the-counter anti-thrush medication. However, if you have CFS it is inadvisable to take these until you are well into recovery as the die-off from the candida that results can set the person back considerably. For this reason it is best to approach the question of anti-candida supplements with a qualified nutritionist to help you. For a full description of available supplement options see *Banish Bloating* in this series of books.

**Heavy metals and pollutants** Toxic elements from our diet, water and environment continually bombard us, and for the most part we can deal with them. However, if we are overwhelmed by these pollutants then a wide variety of health problems can ensue. This is of particular concern to the person with CFS, as their system is already weakened, and these toxic elements may be significantly contributing to the problem. The most obvious and easy steps to take are to eat organic food, to filter water and to avoid fluoride in dental products. Everyday life also exposes us to a number of heavy metals, including lead and copper from water pipes, cadmium from cigarette smoke, mercury from amalgam fillings, fluoride from non-stick pan coatings and aluminium from certain medications, anti-perspirants and foil. To test if you have overly high levels of any of these metals in your body it is best consult a qualified nutritionist who can arrange for a hair sample to be sent to a laboratory (do not be tempted to send off for the hair test often advertised at the back of health magazines).

**Activity** While it is fine to pace yourself by taking a rest when you feel you need it, it is generally agreed that prolonged stays in bed are not helpful for people with CFS. Nevertheless, it must be recognised that exercise can be exhausting, and that there will be some days when it is difficult to even get out of bed. Gentle stretches, perhaps under the tutelage of a physiotherapist, leading to a programme of slowly increased activity, can be of enormous benefit. Fear of the rebound effects of exercise may be sufficient to make you avoid gentle exercise, but it is necessary to overcome this. One study showed that CFS patients had the same level of activity as multiple sclerosis patients, but that the 'cognitive' aspects, in other words what was going on in the minds of sufferers of CFS in terms of anticipated problems, played a much greater part.

## VITAMIN AND MINERAL SUPPLEMENTS

It is generally considered, amongst natural health therapists, that people with CFS probably have multiple nutrient deficiencies. A great many nutrients are needed to support the immune system, particularly when it is under attack, and any deficiency can weaken the immune 'army'.

Most of the important nutrients are covered in **Boost In A Bottle**, page 97, however there are some that are particularly relevant for those with CFS. Vitamin B12 may be of special importance. Sublingual drops are the most absorbable and get around the problem that people with CFS may have reduced intrinsic factor secretion (the element in our digestive tract which allows us to use B12). Some studies have shown that magnesium levels can be low in CFS patients, and the symptoms of magnesium deficiency are very similar to those for chronic fatigue. Other important nutrients for sufferers of CFS are vitamin E and CoQ10.

These are some more specific supplements which can also make a difference:

**Astragalus** This is a potent immune stimulant and it seems to increase white blood cell activity significantly. Research has shown that it is protective against various viruses. It also appears to have the ability to improve tolerance to various stresses, including physical activity.

**NADH** Deficiency of ATP, the cellular energy storing molecule, large stores of which are found in the heart and brain cells, has been linked to severe fatigue, muscle weakness and muscle pain. Early trials have shown that NADH (nicotinamide adenine dinucleotide) can replenish depleted cellular stores of ATP and in this way improve fatigue and cognitive dysfunction. Enada NADH is a stabilised, tablet-form of NADH that is able to clear the digestive tract. It seems to normalise levels of the stress hormone noradrenaline, and some neurotransmitters, including serotonin. It is not useful for relieving muscle pain, but helps to clear the brain. The amounts used in research are 10 mg daily. Supplements are generally 5 mg, but anecdotal evidence is that doses as low as 1 mg can be beneficial. Some long-term users (three years) have found that taking the supplements on alternate days is just as helpful as taking it daily.

**Liquorice root and Ginseng** Both of these can help to stabilise blood sugar and improve low blood pressure problems (so do not take them if you have high blood pressure). In order to achieve the blood pressure elevating/normalising effect you need to use liquorice that contains glycyrrhizin rather than the DGL version (deglycyrrhized). Liquorice root works by stopping the conversion of active adrenal hormones to inactive forms. This results in higher cortisol levels, and can mean greater resistance to the aches and pains of joints and muscles and soft tissue (also called fibromyalgia) suffered by many people with CFS. It can also help recovery from activity, including exercise.

The various ginsengs are also adaptogens which can improve energy and reduce the harmful effects of stress. A useful programme is to start by taking liquorice root for four to six weeks, and then to introduce an adaptogen such as Asian ginseng (100 mg daily standardised extract), Siberian ginseng (300 mg daily standardised extract) or astragalus. While the liquorice root helps to 'jump-start' the adrenal function by improving cortisol levels, the adaptogens then provide support for normal HPA (hypothalamus-pituitary-adrenal) axis feedback. If improvements are noticed at around eight weeks, begin to phase out the liquorice over the next two weeks until you eventually stop it. The ginsengs are best taken for about four weeks, followed by a break of one to two weeks before repeating the cycle. You can also find compounds which combine liquorice and Siberian ginseng. Ginseng should not be overused as it can lead to over-stimulation and insomnia, a particular risk if it is taken with sources of caffeine. It should also not be used by those with high blood pressure, or by women who are pregnant or breastfeeding.

**Milk thistle** This is one of the most widely prescribed herbs by medical doctors in Germany. It plays a specific role in preventing damage to the liver, the organ of detoxification, and has been shown to reverse conditions such as sclerosis of the liver. In conditions such as CFS, given that many sufferers are thought to have compromised immune systems caused by toxic overload, it is important to support the liver actively, to enable it to metabolise food and deal with toxins more effectively.

## ENERGY FIELDS

Energy is an intangible force. We can break down the process by which it is made, and explain what goes into creating energy on a physical level, but not much more than that. Mystics from the earliest times have sought to understand how we derive energy from our surrounding universe, but we are no nearer to knowing the answer.

The main thrust of this book has been to look at chemical energy, since this is generally the starting point for those whose energy generating mechanisms have failed them, usually as a consequence of not providing the basic materials for energy manufacture. In addition, I have touched on the subject of physical energy, which is the sum total of strength, suppleness and stamina generated from the right sort of exercise for a person's constitution.

There are two other types of energy – mental energy and universal energy. Channelling and conserving mental energy is one of the most useful tools, and is a discipline in its own right. The favourite descriptive phrase these days is 'stress management', but it is more than this and entails being the master of your mind rather than being obeisant to it. Tapping into universal energy is the province of spiritualism and religion, but it also plays a part in Chinese medicine and meditation practices.

Stress management, time management, relaxation and/or meditation are not for everybody, but they can be a way of maximising your energy levels and nurturing yourself on every level. Of course, after you have put the information in this book into practice, you may surprise yourself by needing less of these other disciplines than you previously thought. By eating in tune with your body's needs you will find that your moods are less volatile, that you have a less addictive nature, and that your body responds to stress more effectively. In short, you will find you have more energy. Use that energy creatively and wisely. Studies have shown that older people who do 40 hours of charity work a year significantly improve their longevity – which just shows that there is more to optimal health than taking handfuls of vitamins and minerals. It is the complete picture that counts, and being rounded in your view of the world, happy with your own company and generally positive in your outlook can lead to significant improvements in your energy levels.

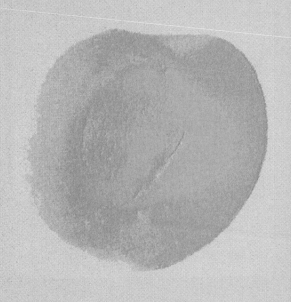

# Part Six

# APPENDICES

# 'Hidden' Sugar in Food

| | Portion | gms | Sugar gms* |
|---|---|---|---|
| chocolate biscuit | 2 biscuits | 15 | 7 |
| digestive biscuit | 1 biscuit | 15 | 2.5 |
| chocolate digestive | 1 biscuit | 15 | 4 |
| rich tea | 2 biscuits | 20 | 4.5 |
| tinned fruit (added sugar) | 1/2 small can | 100 | 23 |
| fruit yoghurt | 1 sml carton | 150 | 14 |
| jam | 2 tsp | 15 | 10.5 |
| mincemeat | 2 tsp | 20 | 12 |
| ice cream | 1 scoop | 50 | 8 |
| cornflakes | 3 tbsp | 30 | 2 |
| sugar puffs | 3 tbsp | 30 | 17 |
| muesli | 1.5 tbsp | 30 | 6 |
| tinned tomato soup | 1/2 tin | 200 | 5 |
| packet tomato soup | 1/4 packet | 20 | 7 |
| baked beans | 1/2 med tin | 225 | 10 |
| tinned sweetcorn | 1/3 tin | 100 | 7.2 |
| Ovaltine | 5 tsp | 16 | 5 |
| orange squash | 1 gls (diluted) | 40 ml | 11.5 |
| cola | 1 can | 300 ml | 32 |
| Ribena | 1 gls (diluted) | 40 ml | 24 |
| ketchup | 2 tsp | 10 | 2 |
| milk chocolate | small bar | 50 | 26 |
| dark chocolate | small bar | 40 | 26 |
| mints | 1 sml tube | 30 | 30 |

* 1 rounded teaspoon of sugar = 5 gms

# Glycaemic Index (GI)

Scientists have so far measured the GI of around 300 high carbohydrate foods. In the US, the measure against which foods are compared is white bread – because it is thought to represent of the type of food usually eaten – which is given a score of 100. In the UK, the measure against which foods are compared is glucose, since this is the sugar that is found in blood, and this is given a score of 100. If converting US figures to UK figures, the US score needs to be multiplied by 0.7. The chart opposite gives the UK figures.

When tested, the amount of food used is that which gives 50 grams of carbohydrate. In practice, this means that some foods need to be eliminated. For instance, you would need to eat an implausibly large amount of celery in order to consume 50 grams of carbohydrate!

It is important to remember that a scoring system such as this gives averages for foods, and for the study participants' reactions to it. The reality is that people have different individual responses to foods, so at best this is a guide. Ideally, you will become sufficiently aware of your response to foods to understand if certain foods are high or low GI for you. Finally, if two foods containing equal amounts of carbohydrate are combined, the GI is the average of the two.

# CEREAL GRAINS

| | | | |
|---|---|---|---|
| barley, pearl | 31 | rice, white, high amylose | 58 |
| rye | 34 | couscous | 65 |
| wheat kernels | 41 | barley, rolled | 66 |
| bulgur | 48 | taco shells | 68 |
| barley, cracked | 50 | cornmeal | 69 |
| buckwheat | 55 | millet | 71 |
| sweetcorn | 55 | tapioca, boiled with milk | 81 |
| rice, speciality | 55 | rice, low amylose | 88 |
| rice, brown | 55 | rice, instant boiled 6 minutes | 90 |
| rice, wild | 57 | | |

## BREADS

| | | | |
|---|---|---|---|
| oat bran bread | 47 | barley flour bread | 66 |
| mixed grain bread | 48 | wheat bread, high fibre | 68 |
| pumpernickel | 50 | wheat bread, wholemeal | 69 |
| bulger bread | 52 | melba toast | 70 |
| linseed rye bread | 52 | bagel, white | 72 |
| pitta bread, white | 58 | wheat bread, white | 78 |
| hamburger bun | 61 | wheat bread, gluten free | 90 |
| rye flour bread | 64 | French baguette | 95 |

## PASTA

| | | | |
|---|---|---|---|
| spaghetti, protein enriched | 27 | linguine | 42 |
| vermicelli | 35 | instant noodles | 47 |
| spaghetti, wholemeal | 37 | spaghetti, durum | 55 |
| ravioli, durum, meat filled | 39 | gnocchi | 67 |
| macaroni | 49 | rice pasta, brown | 92 |

## BAKERY PRODUCTS

| | | | |
|---|---|---|---|
| cake, sponge | 46 | croissant | 67 |
| cake, pound | 47 | crumpet | 69 |
| pastry | 59 | doughnut | 76 |
| muffins | 62 | waffles | 76 |

## BREAKFAST CEREALS

| | | | |
|---|---|---|---|
| rice bran | 19 | Shredded Wheat | 69 |
| All-bran | 42 | Kelloggs Mini-wheats | |
| Bran Buds | 52 | (blackcurrant) | 69 |
| Special K | 54 | wheat biscuit | 70 |
| oat bran | 55 | sultana bran | 71 |
| Kelloggs Honey Smacks | 55 | puffed wheat | 74 |
| muesli | 56 | Cheerios | 74 |
| Kelloggs Mini-wheats | 57 | corn bran | 75 |
| Kelloggs Just Right | 59 | Total | 76 |
| porridge (oatmeal) | 61 | rice crispies | 82 |
| Nutri-grain | 66 | Teams | 82 |
| Grapenuts | 67 | cornflakes | 83 |
| Sustain | 68 | | |

## BISCUITS

| | | | |
|---|---|---|---|
| oatmeal biscuits | 55 | arrowroot biscuits | 67 |
| rich tea | 55 | vanilla wafers | 77 |
| digestives | 59 | morning coffee | 79 |
| shortbread | 64 | | |

## CRACKERS

| | | | |
|---|---|---|---|
| high fibre rye crispbreads | 65 | rice cakes | 77 |
| stone wheat thins | 67 | puffed crispbread | 81 |
| water biscuits | 71 | | |

## DAIRY

| | | | |
|---|---|---|---|
| yoghurt, low fat, artificially sweet | 14 | milk custard | 43 |
| | | Yakult | 45 |
| milk, full fat | 27 | ice cream | 61 |
| milk, skimmed | 32 | | |
| yoghurt, low fat, fruit sugar sweetened | 33 | | |

## FRUIT AND FRUIT PRODUCTS

| | | | |
|---|---|---|---|
| cherries | 22 | grapefruit juice | 48 |
| grapefruit | 25 | orange juice | 52 |
| apricots, dried | 31 | kiwi fruit | 53 |
| pear, fresh | 37 | banana | 54 |
| apple | 38 | fruit cocktail | 55 |
| plum | 39 | mango | 56 |
| apple juice | 41 | sultanas | 56 |
| peach, fresh | 42 | apricots, fresh | 57 |
| orange | 44 | pawpaw | 58 |
| pear, canned | 44 | apricots, canned in syrup | 64 |
| grapes | 46 | raisins | 64 |
| pineapple juice | 46 | pineapple | 66 |
| peach, canned | 47 | watermelon | 72 |

## VEGETABLES

| | | | |
|---|---|---|---|
| carrots | 49 | swede | 72 |
| yam | 51 | chips | 75 |
| sweet potato | 54 | pumpkin | 75 |
| sweetcorn | 55 | potato, instant | 83 |
| potato, new | 57 | potato (old), baked | 85 |
| potato, King Edward, boiled | 63 | carrots, cooked | 85 |
| beetroot | 64 | parsnips | 97 |
| potato, boiled or mashed | 70 | | |

## LEGUMES

| | | | |
|---|---|---|---|
| soya beans, canned | 14 | pinto beans, canned | 45 |
| lentils, red | 18 | baked beans, canned | 48 |
| lentils, green | 29 | peas, green | 48 |
| butter beans | 31 | kidney, beans | 52 |
| split peas, yellow, boiled | 32 | lentils, green | 52 |
| butter beans, baby, frozen | 32 | broad (fava) beans | 79 |
| chickpeas, canned | 42 | | |

## SOUPS

| | | | |
|---|---|---|---|
| tomato soup | 38 | black bean soup | 64 |
| lentil soup, canned | 44 | green pea soup, canned | 66 |
| split pea soup | 60 | | |

## SUGARS

| | | | |
|---|---|---|---|
| fructose | 22 | corn syrup | 62 |
| fruit preserve, no sugar added | 25 | sucrose | 64 |
| lactose | 45 | glucose | 100 |
| jam | 55 | maltodextrin | 105 |
| honey | 58 | maltose | 105 |

## SNACKS

| | | | |
|---|---|---|---|
| peanuts | 15 | popcorn | 55 |
| 70% cocoa solids chocolate | 22 | Mars Bar | 64 |
| Mars M&Ms | 32 | Mars Skittles | 69 |
| Mars Snickers Bar | 40 | corn chips | 74 |
| Mars Twix | 43 | jelly beans | 80 |
| jams and marmalades | 49 | pretzels | 81 |
| chocolate | 49 | dates | 99 |
| potato crisps | 54 | | |

## BEVERAGES

| | | | |
|---|---|---|---|
| soya | 30 | Fanta | 68 |
| cordial, orange | 66 | Lucozade | 95 |

# Resources

To find out more about Suzannah Olivier's activities see her website at:
www.healthandnutrition.co.uk EMAIL: eattobefit@aol.com

## HERBAL AND NUTRIENT SUPPLEMENT SUPPLIERS

**BIOCARE**   Birmingham  Tel: 0121 433 3727
- Stocked by good independent health food shops. Direct mail ordering service available.
- nutrients: large range of vitamins, minerals and essential fats
- blood sugar regulation: Sucroguard
- brain health: Ginkgo Plus
- others: AD 206 for adrenal gland support, TH 207 for thyroid support, CoQ10, Iron EAPZ and Beetroot extract

**BLACKMORES**
- Available from good quality health food shops. A full range of good quality herbs and nutrients for every need.

**HEALTH PLUS**   East Sussex  Tel: 01323 492096
- Supply convenient daily dose packs, each containing a combination of supplements that are designed for specific health conditions. There are 28 daily packs in each box.
- nutrients: range of nutrients

**HIGHER NATURE**   East Sussex  Tel: 01435 882880
- Direct mail-ordering service available. In addition to the products listed below, they also supply flaxseed oil and essential balance oil, which are excellent alternatives to salad oils.
- nutrients: range of vitamins, minerals and essential fats
- blood sugar control:
- brain power: 'Brain Food', ginkgo biloba, phosphatidyl serine
- sleep: serotone (5HTP)
- others: L-glutamine, CoQ10 (Ultra Food Form)

**LAMBERTS**   Kent  Tel: 01892 552120
- Available from health clinics and pharmacies.
- nutrients: large range of vitamins, minerals (including Iron Amino Acid Complex) and essential fats

• • • • • • • • • • • • • • • • • • • • • • • • • • • • • • • • • • •

- blood sugar control: Normoglycaemia®
- brain power: ginkgo biloba
- others: L-glutamine, L-carnitine, high potency royal jelly, CoQ10

**SIMMONDS HERBAL SUPPLIES**  East Sussex  Tel: 0800 542 5212
www.herbalsupplies.com

- A good range of herbal products available by mail order, including ginseng and valerian.

**NUTRI LTD**  High Peak  Tel: 0800 212742

- nutrients: comprehensive range of vitamins, minerals and essential fats
- blood sugar control: GTF complex
- brain power: ginkgo biloba
- others: CoQ10

**THE NUTRI CENTRE**  7 Park Crescent, London W1N 3HE
Tel: 020 7436 5122

- Suppliers of the NutriWest and Health Comm product ranges.
- Stock an extensive range of nutrition products, including NADH, health foods and books from various suppliers and manufacturers. You can either visit the shop or obtain their products by mail order.

**SOLGAR**  Herts  Tel: 01442 890355

- Stocked by good independent health food shops.
- nutrients: large range of low to high dose vitamins, minerals and essential fats and herbs.
- blood sugar control: glucose factor tablets
- brain power and sleep: L-glutamine, Brain Modulator, valerian
- others: L-carnitine, alphalipoic acid, Energy Modulator, Siberian, Korean and American Ginseng, CoQ10, kava kava, rhodiola, ashwagandha.

**FSC**  Tel: 020 8477 5358

- Available from independent health food shops, GNC and Diet Centres.
- ENADA is a stable and absorbable form of NADH. They also have a full range of other good quality supplements.

**PASSION FOR LIFE**  Tel: 0800 096 1121 (mail order)
www.passionforlife.com

- Snorenze (anti-snoring spray) and other useful products.

## NUTRITIONAL THERAPISTS

### BRITISH ASSOCIATION OF NUTRITIONAL THERAPISTS
**(BCM BANT)**  London WC1N 3XX  Tel: 0870 6061284
For a list of registered nutrition therapists please send a large SAE to BANT at the above address.

**INSTITUTE FOR OPTIMUM NUTRITION (ION)** Blades Court, Deodar Road, London SW15 2NU Tel: 020 8877 9993
For a directory of nutritionists, send £2 to the above address.

**BRITISH SOCIETY FOR ALLERGY AND ENVIRONMENTAL MEDICINE (BSAENM)** Southampton Tel: 023 8081 2124
For a list of medical doctors who have a particular interest in nutritional medicine.

**SOCIETY FOR THE PROMOTION OF NUTRITIONAL THERAPY** PO Box 626, Woking, GU22 0XD Tel: 01483 740 903 (answerphone)
For information please send an SAE and £1 to the above address.

## SUPPORT GROUPS AND INFORMATION

**ME ASSOCIATION** Stanhope House, High Street, Standford le Hope, Essex SS17 0HA Tel: 01375 642 466 Information line (Mon-Fri, 1.30-4pm) 01375 361013

**ACTION FOR ME** Information line: 0891 122976

**CFS FOUNDATION** 52 St Enoch Square, Glasgow G1 4AA
Send an SAE for information.

**SAD ASSOCIATION** PO Box 989, Steyning BN44 3HG
Send £5 payable to SADA for an information pack.

**ASH** Website: www.ash.org.uk Tel: 0800 169 0691
For advice about giving up smoking or to speak to a counsellor.

**QUIT** Website: www.quit.org.uk

## USEFUL WEBSITES

**www.mendosa.com**
Gives a useful run down of the whole GI issue and links in to around twenty-five other relevant and useful sites.

**http://easyweb.easynet.co.uk/karenk/recipe.html**
For ideas and recipes for raw foods and dehydrated foods, plus links to other sites.

## BIOCHEMICAL TESTING

Most of these tests are only available through practitioners. If you do obtain one that is available direct to the public, you are strongly advised to have any results interpreted by a nutritionist or other health professional so that they can be acted upon appropriately.

**DIAGNOSTECH LTD** Swansea Tel: 0800 731 5655

Adrenal stress index test which measures the balance of two stress hormones.

**GREAT SMOKIES DIAGNOSTIC LABORATORY**

Tests for adrenal stress, candida, parasites, leaky gut, which can be organised through their UK agents:

Diagnostic Services Ltd Tel: 0151 922 6200

Health Interlink Ltd Tel: 01582 794 094

**THE INDIVIDUAL WELLBEING DIAGNOSTIC LABORATORY**

London SW3 Tel: 020 7730 7010

Tests include allergy and food additive intolerance (FACT), adrenal stress index, Epstein-Barr virus, candida. They run a clinic as well as a postal service. All tests are supported by a nutrition consultation.

## ORGANIC FOOD SOURCES

**THE SOIL ASSOCIATION** Bristol House, 40-56 Victoria Street, Bristol BS1 6BY Tel: 0117 929 0661

The Soil Association provides a list of organic suppliers in the UK, as well as publications on organic issues. Telephone to check the price of the catalogue.

## EQUIPMENT SUPPLIERS

**WHOLISTIC RESEARCH COMPANY** Tel: 01707 262 686

www.holisticresearch.com

A full range of equipment, including water treatment, sprouting jars, juicers and dehydrators, all by mail order.

**HIGHER NATURE** Tel: 01435 882880

Water distillers and supplements.

**AQUAPURE DISTILLATION** Tel: 020 8892 9010

**FRESHWATER FILTER COMPANY** Tel: 020 8558 7495

**THE FRESHWATER COMPANY** Tel: 0345 023998

www.freshwateruk.com

Delivery service in the south east of England of pre-distilled water.

**THE NATURAL ALARM CLOCK** Tel: 01954 211 955

## BOOKS

**Chronic Fatigue Unmasked** Gerald E. Poesnecker, Humanitarian Publishing Co USA (1994)

**Seasonal Affective Disorder** Angela Smyth, Thorsens (1991)

**The Only Way to Stop Smoking Permanently** Alan Carr, Penguin (1995)

**The Stress Protection Plan** Suzannah Olivier, Collins & Brown (2000)

### Diet and Recipe Books

**Cooking Without** Barbara Cousins, Thorsons (1997)

**Optimum Nutrition Cookbook** Patrick Holford and Judy Ridgeway, Piatkus (1999)

**The Sprouter's Handbook** Edward Cairney, Argyll (1997)

**Dry It, You'll Like It** Cauldron, MacManiman and Macmaniman (USA) Available from Wholistic Research Co 01707 262 686

**Superjuice** Michael Van Straten, Mitchell Beazley (1999)